MIGRAINE AND OTHER HEADACHES

MIGRAINE AND OTHER HEADACHES

————

JAMES W. LANCE, M.D.

CHARLES SCRIBNER'S SONS
NEW YORK

To the late Margaret Kendall, my secretary and personal assistant for eighteen years, for her devotion to neurology and headache research

Charles Scribner's Sons
Macmillan Publishing Company
866 Third Avenue, New York, NY 10022
Collier Macmillan Canada, Inc.

Library of Congress Cataloging-in-Publication Data
Lance, James W. (James Waldo)
  Migraine and other headaches.

  Bibliography: p.
  Includes index.
  1. Headache—Popular works.   2. Migraine—Popular
works.   I. Title.   [DNLM: 1. Headache. 2. Migraine.
WL 344 L246m]
RB128.L37   1986   616.8'57   86-3733
ISBN 0-684-18654-3

Originally published under the title
Headache: Understanding Alleviation

Macmillan books are available at special discounts for bulk purchases for sales promotions, premiums, fund-raising, or educational use. For details, contact:

            Special Sales Director
            Macmillan Publishing Company
            866 Third Avenue
            New York, NY 10022

First Paperback Edition 1986

10   9   8   7   6

Designed by Marek Antoniak

Printed in the United States of America

ACKNOWLEDGMENTS

I am indebted to Deborah Carmicael and Patricia Miller for their help in preparing the manuscript. The figures were drawn by Franca Rubiu and Edwina Bates and photographed by the Department of Medical Illustration, University of New South Wales, Sydney.

I am grateful to William Collins & Co. Ltd., London, for permission to quote from James Jones' *The Ice-Cream Headache and Other Stories*; to Robert Hale, London, for permission to quote from Ward McNally's book *Smithy: The Kingsford Smith Story*; to W. B. Saunders and Co., Philadelphia, for permission to quote from *Psychosomatic Medicine* by E. Weiss and O. S. English (3rd ed., 1957); to Ciba-Geigy Ltd., Basel, for permission to reproduce the illustrations by Dr. F. Netter (Figures 7.1, 10.2).

Some of the material is based on my book for medical readership, *The Mechanism and Management of Headache*, 4th edition (London: Butterworths, 1982), from which figures 1.3, 4.2, 5.1, 7.2, 8.4, 8.5, and 9.5 are reproduced by courtesy of the publisher.

The research on which this book is based was made possible by grants from the National Health and Medical Research Council of Australia, the J. A. Perini Family Trust, the Adolf Basser Trust, the Australian Brain Foundation, Sandoz (Australia), Sandoz AG (Basel), and Reckitt and Colman (Australia).

It is impossible to acknowledge adequately my colleagues in neurology and other branches of medicine in many parts of the world whose ideas have influenced those expressed in this book. Truly we all see farther by standing on the shoulders of those who have gone before.

CONTENTS

INTRODUCTION

Migraine is a common and distressing disorder. It is not likely to take life but can destroy the quality of life at what might have been its most rewarding moments. Some 10 percent of men and 20 percent of women suffer from migraine headaches at some time in their lives. If we take the lower of these figures, there should be in excess of 20 million people in the United States alone who stand to benefit from reading this book.

Not all headaches are migraine. The object of this book is to help readers identify their particular headache problem, to discuss what is known about the causes of each type of headache, and then to point the way to preventing headaches by collaboration between headache sufferers and their doctors.

The present text is based on the first edition of this book published by Charles Scribner's Sons in 1975. Knowledge has advanced so rapidly in the past ten years that half the text has had to be rewritten and the remainder revised. The book is written for people without any medical background and should be fairly easy reading, although chapters 2 and 6 may be hard going in places. A glossary and references are placed at the end of the book for those who wish to pursue matters further. Numbers in parentheses in the text indicate the reference on which any particular statement is based. Readers who require more detail may refer to my earlier textbook *The Mechanism and Management of Headache*, 4th edition (London: Butterworths, 1982).

MIGRAINE AND OTHER HEADACHES

1

WHAT KIND OF HEADACHE DO I HAVE?

What Kinds Are There?

There are some lucky people who have never had a headache in their lives and are quite smug about it. Why they should be so blessed, no one knows. It is probably linked with our inheritance of chemical transmitters that pass on messages in the brain from one nerve cell to another. The brain has a control mechanism for pain impulses (see chapter 2), and the transmitter substances involved in this also play a part in the emotions. As a general rule, happy people have fewer headaches than sad people, but this is not the whole answer.

"Normal" Headaches

Many of us get a hangover headache after a late night and a lot of alcohol. Some people are very sensitive to cold, heat, or the glare of sunlight. About one-third of the normal population experiences a sharp pain in the front of the head immediately after swallowing ice cream or a very cold drink. This is usually felt in the center of the forehead (see Figure 1.1) but is sometimes experienced in one temple. An occasional individual has a reaction to certain foods such as salami, hot dogs, or wonton soup. Some drink too much coffee and get rebound headaches as the effect of caffeine wears off. Others get headaches with exercise or even during sexual intercourse. These are described as "normal" headaches in chapter 3, although probably no form of headache should be regarded strictly as normal.

3

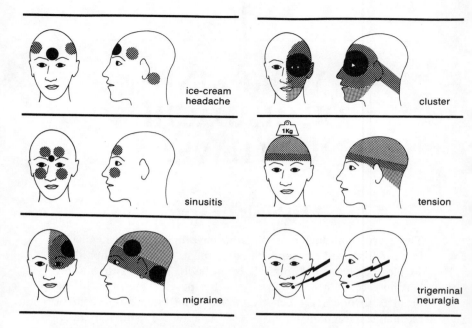

1.1 *What part of the head aches? Regions commonly affected by six varieties of head pain are illustrated; the most severe pain is shown as a concentrated black spot, moderate pain as crosshatched areas, and milder pain or pressure as dotted areas.*

Tension Headache

The times when most of us get a headache are stress-related —at the end of a long, hard day with lots of decisions to be made, lots of talking and listening, and the telephone constantly ringing. This form of tension headache is clearly related to the circumstances that provoke it. There is another form, chronic tension headache (see chapter 8), that persists relentlessly, day after day, as a constant feeling of pressure on or band around the head; it is not always linked with any external situation, although it may be associated with a state of mental depression. Every week or so the headache may increase in severity and throb in time with the pulse, which suggests that blood vessels have become sensitive to pain. This adds an extra component to the headache. This is called a tension-vascular headache and may have some of the characteristics we associate with migraine. It is possible that there is a spectrum of headache, with the chronic tension variety at one end and classical migraine at the other (32). Let us first consider migraine, and then see whether we can draw a clear dividing line between it and tension headache.

Migraine

Classical migraine is easily recognized because it is preceded by visual disturbance. This may consist of little specks or flashes of light that appear in front of the eyes, blurred eyesight, or a more complicated pattern of zigzags that moves slowly across the field of vision for twenty or thirty minutes. As this subsides, aching starts in the front or back of the head, usually on one side only, and becomes progressively more severe. The victims feel sick and may vomit. Light hurts their eyes; they may retire to a dark room and try to sleep it off.

Common migraine is harder to diagnose with certainty because there is no warning sign of disordered vision. The headache may come on in the early hours of the morning and awaken the subject, or it may come on at any other time of the day. It usually (but not always) involves only one side of the head and usually (but not always) is accompanied by nausea and aversion to light. Because there is no one symptom of common migraine that occurs in every attack, it is difficult to distinguish milder episodes from the upsurge of tension headache that we call tension-vascular headache. In fact, it may be artificial to separate these types of headache, for they may be manifestations of the same basic disturbance. The less frequent and more severe the headache, the more likely it is to have the characteristics of migraine (see Figure 1.2). The more frequent the headache, the more likely it will be of a milder form, involving both sides of the head and not associated with nausea and aversion to light. Tension headache can be likened to migraine "drawn out thin," so that some sensation of pressure or discomfort is felt every day. Migraine is like a more severe tension headache bunched up into attacks, alternating with periods of relative freedom from headache. The many variations on the

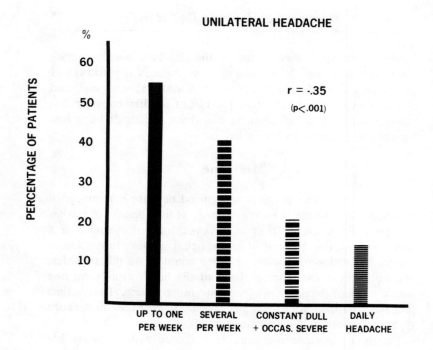

UNILATERAL HEADACHE

%

PERCENTAGE OF PATIENTS

r = -.35
(p<.001)

UP TO ONE PER WEEK • SEVERAL PER WEEK • CONSTANT DULL + OCCAS. SEVERE • DAILY HEADACHE

HEADACHE FREQUENCY

1.2 The prevalence of unilateral (one-sided) headaches is shown in relation to the frequency of attacks. Of headaches recurring once a week or less, 55 percent are unilateral. As the frequency of headache increases, more cases involve both sides of the head, until only about 15 percent of daily headaches are unilateral.

theme of migraine are considered in chapter 4, the factors that may trigger off attacks are presented in chapter 5, and current thoughts on the cause of migraine are discussed in chapter 6. There is no form of treatment of migraine that may be considered a cure, just as there is no cure for asthma or many other illnesses. However, most people with this unpleasant and disabling problem can be treated satisfactorily by modern methods (see chapter 7) so that they have fewer and milder attacks, or in many cases no attacks at all, as long as treatment is continued.

Cluster Headache

The term "cluster headache" has been applied to this distinctive syndrome because it tends to recur in bouts or clusters, each lasting for weeks or months, separated by months or years of freedom from headache. During each bout, the headache occurs one or more times daily as a severe pain centered on one eye but often radiating upward to the forehead and temple or downward over the face on the same side. Each pain lasts for ten minutes to two hours or more before subsiding but may return many times in a twenty-four-hour period, often awakening the sufferer at a set time each night. During each attack, the eye on the side of the headache usually reddens and waters, and the eyelid may droop. In a minority of cases, the headache recurs at regular intervals every few days in the manner of migraine without separating into clusters and remissions, but it can still be diagnosed as a cluster headache because of the severe one-sided pain accompanied by eye changes. Unlike migraine and tension headache, cluster headache affects men more than women. Its cause and management are discussed in detail in chapter 9.

Neuralgia

Any ache that arises from a nerve is called neuralgia. The trigeminal nerve supplies the face and the front part of the brain; the occipital nerves supply the back of the head (see chapter 2). Spontaneous discharge of the trigeminal nerve causes sudden, severe stabbing pains in the face, known as trigeminal neuralgia (see chapter 10). This distressing condition, also called tic douloureux, a French term meaning a painful spasm, usually affects older people. The trigeminal nerve can also become infected by the virus of shingles (herpes zoster virus), which causes an unsightly red rash and blisters over one side of the forehead. This is a painful condition, and the pain may persist as "post-herpetic neuralgia," but the chance of this happening is reduced if the acute attack is promptly treated.

Since branches of the trigeminal nerve are responsible for conveying pain sensation from the eye and sinuses, disease of these structures may cause a headache in the center of the forehead (see chapter 10). The source of pain can usually be recognized fairly easily in these cases, but sometimes migraine headache is mistakenly diagnosed as recurrent sinusitis. In both migraine attacks and sinusitis, the nostril often becomes blocked.

The occipital nerves, which mediate pain from the upper neck and back of the head, are also subject to neuralgia. Aching or sudden jabs of pain may radiate from the junction of the skull and neck upward over the back of the head, often associated with some numbness in the area. Degeneration of disks in the neck or a whiplash injury to the neck may also cause pain in this region (see chapter 10).

Serious Headache

Headache, like pain in other parts of the body, can be a danger signal, a warning that something is going wrong. This is more likely to be the case when it starts suddenly in someone who has never before been troubled with headache, or when a previously established headache pattern alters or becomes more severe. This is a sinister pattern of headache that requires immediate investigation by a neurologist. If you are worried about nasty possibilities, read chapters 11 and 12, but also see your doctor soon.

What Can I Deduce from the Site of Headache?

Different kinds of headache affect parts of the head selectively, as illustrated in Figure 1.1, and so give some clue to the type of attack. This is only a guide, for nature enjoys breaking the rules in order to keep the medical profession on its toes.

Ice-cream headache usually occurs midline, but, if the person also suffers from migraine, the ice-cream headache may be felt in the area usually affected by migraine, commonly in one temple, as shown in Figure 1.1.

Sinusitis causes generalized pain in the forehead if the openings into the frontal air sinuses are blocked, in the center of the forehead if entry to the deep air sinuses (sphenoid, ethmoid sinuses) is blocked, and behind the cheekbones if the maxillary sinuses (antrums) are affected. This is explained further in chapter 10.

Migraine may start in the forehead and temple or in the back of the head. Sooner or later it usually extends between these two areas as a band or bar of pain. Other parts of the head are less commonly affected, but the pain may be felt all over one side of the head (and rarely the face) or, in some cases, even over the whole head.

Cluster headache is usually centered on one eye but may radiate over the forehead and temple, backward to the ear and upper neck, or downward to the nostril, cheek, and teeth on that side.

Tension headache is a tightness or pressure of the head that feels as though a band were wound around it, often combined with the sensation of a weight resting on the head.

Trigeminal neuralgia is a severe stabbing pain in the cheek and upper gum or in the jaw and lower gum. Only rarely (5 percent of cases) does it involve the forehead and eye. It can often be triggered by touching the points illustrated in Figure 1.1.

Serious forms of headache, caused by brain tumors or other developing mischief, may be felt on one or both sides of the head, depending on what area of the brain is affected and whether intracranial pressure is raised. These are suspected according to how the headache has evolved (Figure 1.3) rather than where the headache is located, and on its association with other symptoms such as epileptic fits, the progressive impairment of mental ability or the senses of smell, vision, or hearing, or the loss of skilled movements on one side of the body.

What Can I Deduce from the Pattern of Headache?

By the pattern of headache, we mean the frequency with which attacks recur, the duration of each headache, and whether the condition is stable, improving, or becoming worse.

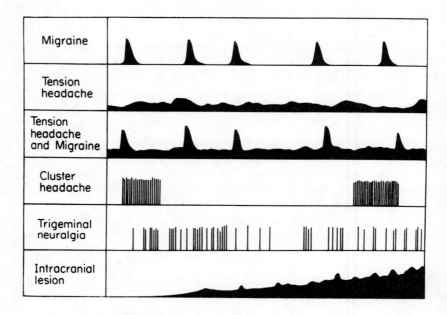

Migraine	
Tension headache	
Tension headache and Migraine	
Cluster headache	
Trigeminal neuralgia	
Intracranial lesion	

1.3 *The different headache patterns develop over a period of time. Migraine is episodic, tension headache relatively continuous, cluster headache recurs in bouts, trigeminal neuralgia recurs irregularly, and headaches caused by intracranial lesions, such as an expanding clot or brain tumor, progressively worsen.*

Migraine headaches are essentially episodic. They may recur irregularly once or twice a year or may follow an established pattern, appearing once a month at the time of menstruation, several times a month, or several times each week (see Figure 1.3). This is in contrast to chronic tension headache, which is usually noticed shortly after awakening and persists throughout the day as an undulating sense of pressure or dullness in the head. The problem of diagnosis is often complicated by the fact that a daily dull headache is punctuated by more severe episodes that resemble migraine (Figure 1.3). This is called combination headache, mixed headache, or tension-vascular headache.

Also illustrated in Figure 1.3 are the habitual bouts of patients suffering from episodic cluster headache, the waxing and waning of pain frequency in trigeminal neuralgia, and the progressive increase in intensity of headache in a patient with a brain tumor or a similar serious structural abnormality. The simple presentation in Figure 1.3 does not actively demonstrate the difference in duration between the pains of trigeminal neuralgia (repeated jabs lasting a fraction of a second) and that of cluster headache (each lasting ten minutes to two hours or more).

One other serious form of headache (not illustrated) is the sudden, explosive onset of headache felt for the first time. This may indeed be an initial episode of migraine but can also be caused by a sudden upsurge of blood pressure or even by the rupture of an intracranial artery spilling blood into the sensitive lining of the brain.

Where Do I Go from Here?

You should now have a general idea of the type of headache that is plaguing you. Fortunately, very few headaches are of grave import or are permanently disabling or life-threatening. Those that are can, for the most part, be successfully treated by the modern techniques outlined in chapters 11 and 12.

The vast majority of recurrent headaches fall into the migraine-tension headache category and can be characterized as enervating, debilitating, and infuriating, but not life-threatening. They can, however, interfere with many of the joys and pleasures of life and with the ability to carry on a normal life at home and at work. If you have identified your particular type of headache from this brief preamble, go on to read the chapters that are relevant to it. Better still, read the entire book, and you will understand much more about yourself, your body, and the way it reacts to produce the most common of all symptoms, headache. You may also find a way to lessen or abolish your headaches and attain one of the most basic of all human rights—freedom from pain.

2

WHY DOES THE HEAD ACHE?

Why Do We Feel Pain?

Headache is a constant or pulsating pain felt in the head. Why do we feel pain at all? Pain is normally a protective device for the body so that any threat of damage can be avoided. If we prick ourselves on a sharp object, we withdraw our hand or foot from it. If we sprain an ankle, pain forces us to rest the joint until it recovers. Pain is caused by impulses that pass along the nerve fibers, like brief electrical discharges. Most nerves in the body can give rise to the sensation of pain if the frequency of discharges within the nerve fibers rapidly increases. For example, touching a warm object with the hand will set up a train of impulses in the nerves passing from the hand to the spinal cord. As the object becomes hotter, the number of impulses each second increases. If heat becomes so great that the skin is in danger of burning, the nerve fires off impulses rapidly and continuously. This burst of activity is then interpreted as pain by the central nervous system.

Some nerve fibers specialize in conveying the message of pain. One group conducts the impulses quite quickly and another very slowly. If we touch a hot stove, we remove our hand immediately because of a sharp, painful sensation. A second or so later another throb of pain is felt as the slower nerve fibers deliver their message to reinforce the first.

The sensation of pain thus serves a useful purpose. It is only when it becomes excessive and persistent that it ceases to be a warning device and becomes an agent of misery. Pain in the head can arise from the nerve fibers responsible for sensation in the scalp, muscles, and bones of the neck and skull. More commonly it comes from arteries that supply the face, scalp, and brain with blood, because the arterial walls contain fine nerve filaments, called a nerve plexus, which are highly sensitive to stretch.

I have heard an occasional person boast that he or she has never experienced a headache and does not know what headache is; at the other end of the spectrum are those unfortunate people who react to commonplace situations by developing a headache. Others are subject to headache without any discernible reason in their life or their surroundings.

Headache is almost entirely subjective. Doctors have to rely on the description of the person who suffers from it to make a diagnosis and assess its severity. For this reason we cannot tell whether animals suffer from headache. It is true that a very severe headache will cause pallor, sweating, nausea, and vomiting, but usually the observer has little guidance other than the subject's own words. Even though everyone lives in his or her own perceptual world, the perception of pain does not differ greatly from person to person.

Pain Threshold

The pain threshold can be measured by a number of standard methods, such as the application of measured amounts of heat to the skin. This threshold has been found to be remarkably consistent, varying for one person only 3 percent from the average value and within a group of two hundred people by no more than 15 percent (114). It appears from all experiments that the pain threshold in humans is fairly stable and bears no consistent relation to age, sex, fatigue, or the normal range of emotions. The threshold can be lowered by a previous injury to a particular area or by sunburning of the skin and can be raised by hypnosis, suggestion, distracting the attention, concentration on other things, and competing stimuli such as acupuncture.

Medications that relieve pain, known as analgesics, can also raise the pain threshold, but so can dummy tablets. Hippocrates pointed out that "of two pains occurring together, not in the same part of the body, the stronger weakens the other" (3). This is the principle of counterirritation, as illustrated in the use of linaments to relieve limb pains or by the application of hot cups to the chest, which produce a partial vacuum as they cool. This traditional treatment for pleurisy is still in vogue in some parts of the world.

While the sensation of pain is much the same in everyone, the reactions to it differ widely. Some of these are reflex reactions and usually not subject to voluntary control, such as alteration of heart rate, blood pressure, and the blood supply to the skin, which controls skin color. When headache is present, there is often a reflex contraction of the muscles of the head and neck, which may give a feeling of stiffness to the neck. Other physical reactions, which are under voluntary control, depend on the cultural background and upbringing of the individual. Some people are much given to expression of their bodily sensations in colorful language and gesticulation. Others may have a more stoic philosophy; their symptoms can be uncovered only by careful questioning. Those who are interested and active in the world around them may suppress the sensation of a mild headache and carry out a normal day's routine. Others who lead a solitary life and are inactive, depressed, or introspective may dwell on their symptoms until their severity becomes progressively magnified. Fear walks hand in hand with pain. If a patient does not understand that a headache is typical of migraine or nervous tension, he or she may be afraid that it is caused by a cerebral tumor or that it could lead to a stroke. The idea of such a disaster grows in the mind until one thinks of little else. Explaining the causes of pain and the natural history of the headache is therefore the first step in coming to terms with the symptoms and helping to overcome them. The more people understand the cause of their headaches, the more calm and relaxed they become, and the more the intensity of the headache is reduced. The less pain one experiences, the more the headache is seen in perspective to the rest of life and the process of relaxation reinforced. What could have been a vicious circle—pain and anxiety spiraling upward together—is converted to a gentle decline of symptoms, with pain and anxiety ultimately subsiding together.

Pain Pathways

Pain from the head and neck comes from the nerves supplying the skin, scalp, muscles, and joints or from the deeper structures, such as the skull and the membranes lining the brain. Curiously enough, the brain itself is insensitive to pain. In fact, some brain operations can be carried out with the patient wide awake. If the surface of the brain, the cortex, is touched or stimulated by an electric current, the patient may feel a tingling down the opposite side of the body, see flashes of light in front of the eyes, or experience other sensations depending on the part of the brain that is stimulated. But the patient does not feel pain even if the brain tissue is cut with a scalpel.

The largest of the nerves, responsible for sensation from the face and for the front two-thirds of the scalp, is called the trigeminal nerve because it has three separate divisions (see Figures 2.1, 2.2). (The Latin *trigeminus* means "three born at a birth.") If this nerve is irritated it causes pain in the forehead, check, or jaw, depending on which of the three divisions is involved. If, for example, sinuses in the forehead are inflamed, the swollen lining of the sinuses compresses the fine nerve branches embedded there. The pressure sets up nerve impulses that travel along the first division of the trigeminal nerve. If the maxillary sinuses (antrums) in the cheekbones or a tooth in the upper jaw become infected, pain is conveyed by the second division. If a tooth in the lower jaw or the jawbone itself is the cause of the trouble, the pain impulses travel in the third division. The three divisions join together inside the skull, where their combined fibers enter the brain stem, which lies under the brain like the stalk of a mushroom (Figures 2.1, 2.2). Some fibers pass directly upward into the brain itself, while others make a loop downward into the upper part of the spinal cord. This loop is of great importance in understanding pain of the head and neck, because it connects with the same nerve

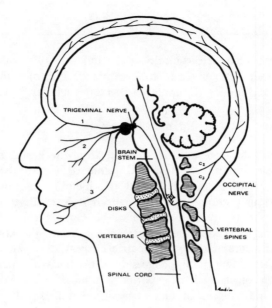

2.1 *The main nerves of the head. Sensation from the front part of the head, the cheek, and the chin is conveyed by the three divisions of the trigeminal nerve (numbered 1, 2, 3). Sensation from the back part of the head travels in the occipital nerves through the second and third cervical spinal nerve roots (labeled C2, C3). Some nerve fibers of both pathways connect with the same cells in the upper part of the spinal cord (designated by the diamond), thus conveying pain arising from the neck to the forehead and vice versa.*

cells that receive impulses from the upper part of the neck. For this reason, a disturbance of the bones or disks in the upper part of the head and neck can cause pain to be felt in the eye and forehead, a phenomenon known as referred pain. When this pathway is operating in the reverse direction, a headache such as migraine can be accompanied by severe pain and stiffness in the neck.

In addition to supplying the face and skull with pain sensation, the trigeminal nerve is responsible for sensations coming from the blood vessels in the brain and scalp. The most common sources of headache are dilatation, distension, and displacement of the blood vessels. When an artery becomes

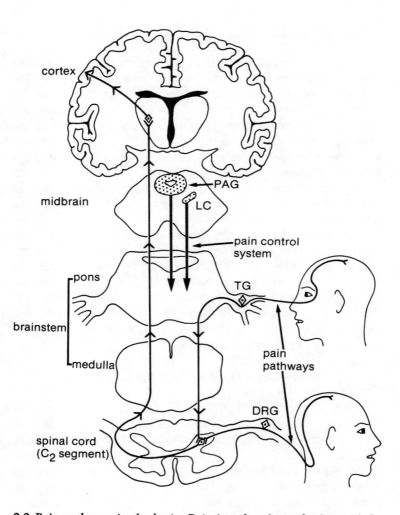

2.2 *Pain pathways in the brain. Pain impulses from the front of the head are conveyed to the trigeminal ganglion (TG) and then to the brain stem, where they descend to the upper spinal cord. Here they synapse on the same cells as fibers coming from the back of the head via the dorsal root ganglion (DRG). After this convergence, the combined pathway crosses to the opposite side and travels upward to the cerebral cortex. The pain-control system projects downward to the brain stem and spinal cord from the periaqueductal gray matter (PAG) and locus ceruleus (LC) to regulate the transmission of pain impulses, as shown in Figure 2.3.*

distended, the delicate network of nerve fibers around it stretches and gives off signals that may increase with each pulse, so the headache may be described as throbbing. The arteries of the scalp contribute to some forms of headache like migraine, and can be felt to pulsate more than usual. Firm pressure over the pulse in front of the ear or over the affected area will diminish the severity of the headache, because less blood flows through the sensitive vessels with each pulse. In other forms of headache, such as hangover, the arteries inside the skull are dilated and sensitive, so that jarring the head or bending the head forward will make the pain worse.

If we draw a line straight upward from the ear, any pain in front of that line results from activity in the trigeminal nerve, and any pain behind the line comes from the spinal nerves that run down over the back of the head to join the upper part of the spinal cord (Figure 2.2). The same spinal nerves supply the lining of the rear of the brain and the brain stem, so that pain felt in the back of the head can arise from inside the skull or from the upper part of the neck.

Passing On the Pain Message

When pain is felt in the forehead or temples, electrical impulses pass along the first division of the trigeminal nerve to the trigeminal ganglion (TG in Figure 2.2), which contains their nerve cells. One branch of these nerve cells brings pain impulses from the head and another branch carries the message to the central nervous system. This central branch plunges downward from the pons through the medulla to the upper part of the spinal cord, the second cervical segment (C2 in Figure 2.2), where it meets the next nerve cell in the pathway. To pass on its message, the nerve fiber releases a chemical substance that excites the second cell. The nature of this chemical is not known with certainty but is thought to be a peptide that has been called "substance P" (SP in Figure 2.3). Once the second nerve cell or neuron is excited, an electrical wave passes through it upward to the brain, where the message is received by the cerebral cortex, the thinking part of the brain (Figure 2.2).

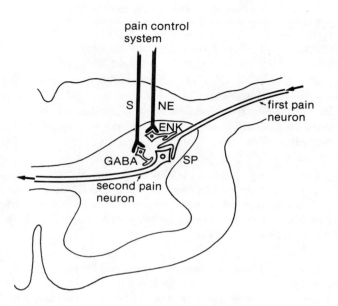

2.3 *The gateway for pain. Transmission of impulses from incoming pain fibers to the next nerve cell depends on the release of substance P (SP), which is controlled by small interneurons releasing enkephalins (ENK) and GABA. These in turn are regulated from the brain stem by the pain-control system, which releases serotonin (S) and norepinephrine (NE). In this way the brain can modulate the perception of pain.*

A similar pathway signals pain from the back of the head by impulses in the occipital nerves (Figure 2.1) that join the second cervical nerve root and connect with their cell bodies in the dorsal root ganglion (DRG in Figure 2.2). Their central branch plunges into the spinal cord at the second cervical segment (Figures 2.1 and 2.2) and excites some of the fibers described above. Although some trigeminal fibers do have their own direct pathway to the brain, many of them share the use of the second pain neuron with the inflow from the back of the head and upper neck. This is a curious but necessary economy of nature, as there is simply not enough room in the brain stem for each nerve cell to have its own direct line to the brain. This principle is commonly observed in the nervous system. Nerve fibers conduct their messages electrically, then converge on nerve cells, where they pass on their message chemically. The point where one nerve cell makes contact with another is known as a synapse, and the chemical mediator is called a neurotransmitter. Transmission at a synapse is controlled by other cells, termed interneurons, that can dampen a nerve cell's activity so that the brain is not flooded by a lot of unneeded information. This is particularly important in the case of pain, since we need to feel just enough to warn us of any mischief going on, but not so much that the sensation of pain is constant. The brain, therefore, has its own pain control system. If this does not function normally we can feel pain spontaneously, one of the factors that produces headache. Let us see how the pain control system works.

How the Brain Controls Pain

Small nerve cells, termed interneurons, sit astride the first junction (synapse) in the pain pathway (Figure 2.3). The interneurons release enkephalin, a naturally occurring substance that acts like morphine. Morphine is prescribed widely by physicians for the relief of severe pain. Enkephalins are also called endorphins, meaning endogenous (occurring inside the body) morphinelike substances. The "high" felt by marathon runners is thought to be caused by the release of endorphins. Morphine is manufactured from opium, so the pain-control chemicals in humans have also been called opioids. If morphine is administered to someone in pain, it binds onto the receptor sites normally used by the body's own opioids and prevents the release of substance P, so as to block the transmission of pain impulses. Under normal conditions enkephalins perform this function. There are other chemical agents released by interneurons. One of these is gamma-aminobutyric acid (GABA), which reduces the excitability of the second neuron in the pathway and thus reduces its response to pain signals. These two agents, enkephalin and GABA, guard the gateway for the entry of pain into the nervous system. These sentinels could not be allowed to act on their own, blocking pain impulses in a whimsical or capricious fashion. They have to obey commands from the brain so that pain messages are admitted when required and halted when irrelevant. Marathon runners must ignore the complaints of joints and muscles in order to finish the race, but afterward want to get the information from their limbs to see how they have stood up to their ordeal.

To adjust the fine tuning of the pain gateway, the brain controls the action of interneurons by nerve pathways that run down from parts of the midbrain (Figure 2.2) to the brain stem and spinal cord (Figure 2.3). One of these areas surrounds the aqueduct, a tube that carries fluid through the midbrain and is known as the periaqueductal gray matter (PAG in Figure 2.2). Another important area is called the locus ceruleus (LC in Figure 2.2), which means "a blue spot" because it appears blue to the naked eye. Nerve fibers from the periaqueductal gray matter release a monoamine serotonin (S) onto the interneurons, while the fibers from the locus ceruleus release another monoamine, norepinephrine (NE). The terminals of these descending pain-control pathways are shown in Figure 2.3, adjusting the action of interneurons so that the brain receives either more or less pain information (9).

What Happens in Headache?

This pain control system is important for understanding headache. We know that the blood levels of monoamines (serotonin and norepinephrine) increase before the onset of migraine headache and then decrease during the headache phase. In chronic tension headache the blood level of serotonin remains low all the time. If these blood levels reflect the action of the same chemicals in the brain, the pain-control pathway would be inactive during headache, so that impulses could flood in from the head and neck to cause constant pain.

Something else is also going on in headache. Blood vessels become sensitive, so that every variation of blood pressure caused by the heartbeat sends off waves of pain impulses from the wall of the blood vessels as they distend. It has been shown that naturally occurring substances such as bradykinin will make blood vessels sensitive if serotonin is applied to the vessels at the same time. Professor Federigo Sicuteri and his team in Florence have shown that the combination of bradykinin and serotonin injected into the veins of human volunteers makes the veins ache (101). Before that, it was known that the same combination applied to the base of a blister was extremely painful.

It looks as though serotonin plays a part in headache in at least two separate ways. It is released into the bloodstream at the onset of headache and is thought to be adsorbed to the blood vessels of the brain and scalp, making them sensitive to pain. Then, when pain impulses arrive at the central nervous system, the normal checking system is broken down because of the lack of serotonin, so that an excessive number of impulses pass through the pain pathways to the brain and give rise to headache.

There are other factors to consider, to be sure, and these will be mentioned as each variety of headache is examined. Nevertheless, grasping the principles outlined in this chapter will give headache sufferers some idea of what is taking place in the nervous system to cause this unpleasant symptom.

3

"NORMAL" HEADACHES

Headaches may be brought on by fairly normal circumstances in some susceptible people, who often are those subject to migraine or related forms of recurrent headache.

Excessive Nerve Stimulation

A constant pressure on the nerves of the scalp, caused even by wearing a tight hat or headband, can cause headache. Queen Mary Tudor, at her coronation, was said to have rested her head on her hand to ease the headache aggravated by her heavy jeweled diadem. More recently there have been reports of "goggle headache" from swimmers wearing tight-fitting goggles that compress the nerves running from the orbit over the forehead. In some instances the pressure from the goggle strap has produced a full-blown migraine attack several hours after training ceased. Such headaches can be prevented by changing the position of the goggles each day or using goggles with a single soft-rubber rim that fits around both ends and does not require a very tight head strap in order to be watertight. Exposure to icy winds or diving into very cold water can cause sudden headache. Eating very cold food can excite the nerves in the mouth and palate enough to cause headache. This has been called "ice-cream headache" and is another example of referred pain.

Ice-Cream Headache

Holding ice or ice cream in the mouth or swallowing it while it is still very cold may cause a localized pain in the palate or throat and sometimes a headache in the forehead or temple because of referred pain from the trigeminal nerve endings. Occasionally it may produce pain behind the ear because this area is supplied by another cranial nerve, the glossopharyngeal, which also has branches over the back of the throat that may be thrown into sudden activity by intense cold. The condition is sufficiently well known to have been used as a title for a collection of short stories, *The Ice-Cream Headache* by James Jones (56). In the title story, referring to the grandfather and his grandchildren, Jones wrote, "He loved to feed them large doses of ice cream on summer afternoons, would laugh at them gently when they got the terrible sharp headaches from eating too much too fast, and then give them a gentle lecture on gluttony."

The condition was mentioned as far back as 1850 in Daniel Drake's *Principal Diseases of North America* (29).

> The consumption of ice cream has been increasing in the Valley, for the last quarter of a century; previously to which its use was quite limited. At present, it is used in summer, in all our cities, from the Lakes to the Gulf of Mexico; and makes an important part of the luxuries provided by the wealthier classes, for their evening parties, throughout the year. For a long time, many persons regarded it as dangerous in hot, and absurd in cold weather; but these prejudices are now nearly extinct. I have not had occasion to observe any injurious effects from it, that might not be traced to two heads: first, swallowing it before the ice has dissolved in the mouth, when it sometimes raises an acute pain in the pharynx, and gives a sense of coldness and sinking in the stomach; second, eating it when the stomach is torpid and inactive from dyspepsia, and the individual is inclined, at the time, to sick headache. The composition, not less than the coldness, contributes to the injury in this case. Under all other circumstances, ice cream may be regarded as equally salubrious and pleasant.

The origin of ice-cream headache is in the roof of the mouth, where sudden cooling occurs. Cooling of the esophagus (the tube that connects the throat with the stomach), or of the stomach itself, does not cause headache. It is interesting that Drake was aware of a connection with "sick headache" (migraine). In San Francisco, Dr. Neil H. Raskin and his colleague, Dr. S. C. Knittle, reported in 1976 that cold drinks or ice cream evoke headache in 93 percent of migrainous patients, compared with only 31 percent of the general population (93). In our own clinic, Dr. Peter Drummond and I found that about one-third of those people suffering from migraine feel their ice-cream headache in the same area as their migraine headache (33). This suggests that the appropriate nerve pathways are very sensitive in migraine sufferers. The more severe and typical the migraine headache, the more likely the patient is prone to ice-cream headache (see Figure 3.1).

Hot-Dog Headache

Other forms of headache result from simple dilatation (expansion) of the blood vessels inside the skull, particularly the intracranial arteries. Continuing the gastronomic line of thought, we can now consider headaches caused by certain foods or chemical substances contained within them. We shall leave the question of foods triggering migraine headache to a later chapter.

Some individuals develop headache shortly after eating hot dogs or other cured-meat foods. Originally rock salt was used in the preparation of cured meats. The patchy appearance of the final product was caused by sodium nitrite, an impurity of the salt. Nitrites are now added to salt in order to produce a uniform red look to the meat. Nitrites are well known as dilators of blood vessels, and, even though the usual concentration of nitrites in cooked meat is only 50 to 130 parts per million, some people are susceptible to headache after eating hot dogs, bacon, ham, or salami.

Dr. William R. Henderson and Dr. Neil H. Raskin studied a man who experienced a moderately severe headache in

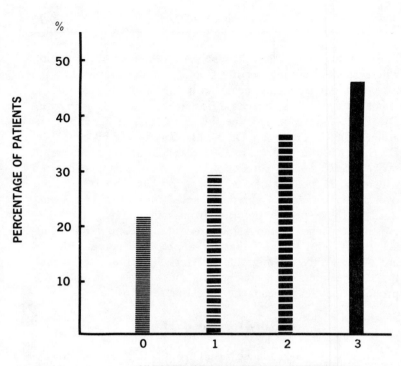

3.1 *Ice-cream headache and migraine. The prevalence of ice-cream headache increases from 20 percent in those patients without migraine to 50 percent in patients who are subject to all three of the symptoms typical of migraine (neurological symptoms, one-sided headache, and nausea). From Drummond and Lance, 1984 (32).*

both temples within thirty minutes of eating cured-meat products (50). The attacks usually lasted for several hours, sometimes acompanied by flushing of the face. The man did not have headaches at other times. It was found that small amounts (10 milligrams) of a solution of sodium nitrite produced a headache eight out of thirteen times, while a solution of sodium bicarbonate of similar taste and appearance had no effect. This particular patient was also sensitive to tyramine, another chemical that will be mentioned later in the chapter on migraine. Normal volunteers did not react to either chemical substance.

The Chinese Restaurant Syndrome

Some unfortunate people experience sensations of pressure and tightness in the face, burning over the trunk, neck, and shoulders, and a pressing pain in the chest after eating a Chinese meal. A few of them also complain of headache—usually those who are susceptible to migraine or other vascular headaches. The headache is a pressure or throbbing over the temples and a bandlike sensation around the forehead, coming on twenty to twenty-five minutes after eating Chinese food and lasting for an hour. Dr. Herbert H. Schaumburg and his colleagues in New York have shown that the offending substance is monosodium L-glutamate (MSG), which is widely used as a food additive, particularly in Chinese cuisine (99). All subjects tested developed the "Chinese restaurant syndrome" if they consumed enough MSG on an empty stomach. Once some other food had been eaten, even the most susceptible did not develop headache. For this reason, soup usually precipitated the headache, as it is consumed before any other food is taken. About three grams of MSG will produce an attack in sensitive individuals. This amount is contained in about 200 milliliters (seven ounces) of wonton soup. The symptoms are caused by the direct action of MSG on blood vessels. Moral: take food before soup in a Chinese restaurant if you are one of the unhappy few.

Hangover

MSG is not the only dilator of blood vessels. Alcohol is a potent dilator, as the flushed appearance of any bon vivant will testify. Patients who are prone to migraine may notice that red wines trigger an attack, but that they can drink white wines without any worry. The histamine content of alcoholic drinks, particularly red wine, was thought to be the culprit, but it is now know that histamine is broken down in the stomach so that very little is absorbed. There are many other substances in alcoholic drinks that could be responsible. Various aldehydes and esters (collectively called congeners) are present in large amounts in beer, port, and table wines, and to a lesser degree in distilled drinks such as whiskey, vodka, and gin. Many patients say that it is safer for them to stick to spirits. The safest choice is not to drink alcohol at all if you are in a susceptible phase of migraine or cluster headache.

Since a hangover is usually a feature of the morning after, it is probably not the direct result of alcohol but rather the effect of its breakdown products (acetaldehyde and acetate), which are then circulating in the bloodstream and cause a painful relaxation of the arteries inside the skull. The added factors of a late night, loud conversation or music, excitement, and possibly nervous tension and cigarette smoking may all contribute to the end result. Remedies that constrict blood vessels, including caffeine in coffee and tea, are helpful, as well as the usual analgesics. Dr. Neil H. Raskin and Dr. O. Appenzeller concluded a review of hangover headache by stating: "The performance of experiments that very often must take place on Sunday mornings may be an important factor in perpetuating our ignorance" (92).

Marijuana

A mild frontal headache may be experienced by users of marijuana. On the other hand, tension headache may be relieved by marijuana, probably because of its relaxing effect.

Fasting Headache

While excess of some foods and drinks can touch off headache, abstaining from food may do the same in some cases. A lowered blood sugar level is a known trigger for migraine, and a dull headache often accompanies any prolonged fast. The chain of events is complex and appears to involve the formation and release of fatty acids into the bloodstream. Just because a headache regularly occurs in the early hours of the morning does not mean that it is caused by low blood sugar. And it is not likely to be prevented by eating before going to bed.

Rebound Headache

Substances such as caffeine, nicotine, and ergotamine constrict blood vessels and therefore diminish any vascular headache. If these substances continually enter the bloodstream, the vessels adapt to a semiconstricted state; they will dilate if the constricting agent is withdrawn, causing headache. The sufferer from tension headache who habitually takes caffeine in tablets or powders in combination with analgesics may develop a headache as the effect wears off. Similarly, a consistently large amount of tea or coffee can lead to a withdrawal headache if the supply is not maintained. Patients who are prescribed ergotamine to ward off a migraine attack are ill advised to take these pills more than once a day. If they do, the chances are that they will prevent one headache only to lay the foundation for the next. This type of headache is called rebound headache because of the cycle of vascular constriction and dilatation. It is probable that smokers' headaches belong to this same category because of the constricting effect of nicotine, although nervous tension may also be partly responsible.

Exertional Vascular Headaches

Now that we have shown that food, alcohol, tea, coffee, and smoking can all play a role in provoking headaches, it seems only fair to incriminate sporting and sexual activities as well. It can be seen that avoidance of all activities that have been known to cause headache can lead to a fairly quiet and unadventurous existence. There is no need to lose heart, however, because these forms of headache are not very common and can be prevented in ways other than a monastic life.

Any form of exercise can precipitate headache in some unfortunate people, and some of its forms are named after the exertion that produces them; for example, "weight-lifter's headache." Many young people have been on the verge of giving up competitive sports because they have invariably developed a throbbing headache after strenuous exertion. Older patients are often unable to finish a day's work of gardening because of headache. In many of these cases the headache could be prevented by taking tablets to constrict the blood vessels of the head before starting the day's exertion. In some cases exercise can also provoke a migraine headache, and this may be prevented in the same way. During exercise, the blood pressure rises, the pulse rate increases, and arteries throughout the body increase in diameter. This process of dilatation normally affects the small vessels as well as the large so that the face becomes flushed and veins stand out on the temple or forehead, indicating that blood is flowing more rapidly through the scalp. The probable cause of headache during exercise is that the smaller vessels do not dilate enough to keep pace with the larger ones, and the face remains pale even though the arteries are distended and pulsating more than usual. The blood in the arteries is under increased pressure because it cannot escape easily through the small channels in skin and muscle. The vessel wall is therefore stretched and gives rise to the sensation of pain. The treatment, which ensures that the arteries do not dilate excessively, is to take ergotamine tartrate or indomethacin (Indocin) before beginning exercise. Another possibility, which may appeal to some, is to give up exercise.

Cough Headache

A variation on exertional vascular headache is a headache felt only when coughing, sneezing, bending, or straining. Sometimes this may be serious, because it may signal an obstruction blocking the flow through the normal fluid channels of the brain, the ventricles. It always warrants a consultation with a doctor. It used to be thought that a cough headache was invariably due to a serious cause until Sir Charles Symonds, a great English neurologist, described twenty-seven patients with cough headache, of whom only six were found to have a brain tumor or similar intracranial abnormality (108). He coined the term "benign cough headache" to describe the symptom of the remaining twenty-one patients, because fifteen of them gradually improved without any treatment. Dr. E. D. Rooke of the Mayo

Clinic studied 103 patients who complained of headache when running, bending, coughing, sneezing, lifting, or straining during a bowel movement (97). This form of headache was more common in men than in women in a proportion of 4:1. After ten years elapsed, seventy-three patients lost their headaches entirely or had greatly improved. A structural abnormality was found in only ten patients during the follow-up period. The outlook for recovery is therefore promising, but it is important that the patient remain under the supervision of a neurologist, who will ensure that the condition is indeed benign cough headache.

Mountain Sickness

Headache is the most frequent complaint of climbers who ascend to high altitudes without oxygen support. It commonly affects both sides of the head, but is limited to one side in about one-quarter of cases. The headache resembles that of migraine and may be prevented in some instances by taking acetazolamide or other drugs that alter salt and fluid balance.

Sexual Intercourse Headache (Benign Sex Headache)

Headache occurring at or near the climax of sexual intercourse is happily uncommon. It may be intensely severe, throbbing or bursting in character. This naturally gives rise to much alarm and apprehension. It is true that the increase in blood pressure which accompanies enthusiastic sexual intercourse may sometimes be of serious import if there is some underlying abnormality in the blood vessels of the brain. In most cases it is simply the result of muscle contraction and a sudden dilatation of the blood vessels in response to an increase in blood pressure. I wonder if Hippocrates had this in mind when he wrote of "immoderate venery" in the fifth century B.C., "One should be able to recognise those who have headache from gymnastic exercises, or running, or walking, or hunting or any other unseasonable labour, or from immoderate venery" (3).

The late Harold G. Wolff, Professor of Neurology, Cornell, New York Hospital, described four patients, all women, aged forty to fifty-six, who experienced sudden severe pain in the head at the beginning of orgasm (114). The headache lasted from several minutes to several days in different instances. In one patient in whom the headache persisted, the opportunity arose to record her blood pressure, which was found to be high. After the blood pressure subsided and the headache disappeared, the patient became emotionally upset. Her blood pressure again shot up, and the same type of headache recurred. It is well known that sudden increases of blood pressure from other causes may also provoke a transient vascular headache.

From my own practice I analyzed the case histories of twenty-five patients with this complaint, nineteen of whom were male and six female, from eighteen to fifty-eight years of age (62). The headache was brought on by sexual intercourse in twenty-one cases, by masturbation alone in one, and by both forms of sexual activity in three. The headache usually comes on gradually as sexual excitement increases, with a feeling of tightness or pressure felt at the back of the head and neck. This is probably caused by excessive contraction of the head and neck muscles, as deliberate relaxation of these muscle groups can bring relief. If sexual activity stops at this point, the headache usually subsides over a period of five minutes to two hours. Those who continue to orgasm often experience a severe generalized headache, explosive and frightening at onset, which persists for two to four hours. This is probably caused by a sudden increase in blood pressure at the climax of sexual activity.

These headaches are more likely to occur if there is an element of nervous tension at the time. One woman described herself as "striving for orgasm" when she was struck by an intensely severe headache. One young man complained of headache at orgasm when he was on vacation, having sexual intercourse two or three times daily. When his holiday was over and the frequency of sexual intercourse declined, the headaches disappeared. Other subjects confirmed that the headache was more likely to come on if they were attempting intercourse for a second time after a brief interval. The headache was not related solely to physical exertion. One man experimented with different techniques to track down the cause of his headache. He found that the headache came on even if he lay on his back and played a completely passive role. There was no physical exertion at all on his part, but he became aware of tension building up in his forehead, jaw, and neck muscles until the headache started about one minute before ejaculation.

Masters and Johnson gave physiological data taken from their studies of the human sexual response that support the views expressed concerning the mechanism of the two components of headache (76). During orgasm, the heart rate increases to 110 to 180 beats per minute, and blood pressure rises by 20 to 80 percent. The cardiovascular changes are just as great during masturbation as in sexual intercourse. Masters and Johnson also comment on muscular contraction, or myotonia. They state: "With plateau phase established, myotonic response is clinically obvious from forehead to toes of the responding individual. In reacting to elevated sexual tension levels, the individual frowns, scowls or grimaces as facial muscles contract involuntarily in semispasm. . . . During automanipulation the jaws frequently are clenched spastically." Again, "The muscles of the neck contract involuntarily in a spastic pattern. As the result, the neck is usually held rigidly in mid-position." It is quite clear that the muscle contraction described is sufficient to initiate the greatest tension headache of all time.

Sex headaches are capricious in that they may develop on several successive occasions and then no longer trouble the person again, without any obvious change in sexual technique. They are not always benign, as several cases have been reported of young men who had a mild stroke at the height of headache, probably caused by spasm of the arteries that supply the brain stem with blood. Because of the occasional vascular complication, anyone experiencing a headache during sexual intercourse is well advised to desist on that particular occasion and consult a doctor.

It remains a mystery as to why the condition suddenly starts at any one particular time, and is not related to the age of the patient. It warrants keeping an eye on the patient's blood pressure, but it is usually a harmless condition that vanishes as suddenly as it appears. It may be prevented by taking certain pills before sexual activity starts, such as ergotamine tartrate (used in the treatment of acute migraine) or propranolol (Inderal), which blocks the action of epinephrine. However, this headache is so unpredictable, occurring on some occasions and not others, that a pharmacological approach hardly seems worthwhile. The term "benign orgasmic cephalgia" seems appropriate, although I would prefer to call it "benign sex headache" in line with "benign cough headache" and similar entities.

Conclusions

Enough has been said to show that a headache may arise in anyone when the nerve supply to the blood vessels or other structures of the head is stimulated excessively. It is important to determine that these headaches are simply an overreaction of normal structures to unusual circumstances and do not indicate any abnormality of these structures or their nerve pathways. The physician is fortunately able to give that reassurance to most patients.

4

WHAT IS MIGRAINE?

Defining the Migraine Syndrome

The concept of migraine as an intermittent headache, sometimes preceded or accompanied by flashing lights in front of the eyes or other disturbances of brain function, was introduced in chapter 1. Although experienced clinicians understand what the term "migraine" means and can recognize it when they see it, it is difficult to provide a definition that will satisfy and educate everybody. The best I can do is say that migraine is episodic headache, cerebral disturbance, or both, with intervening periods of relative freedom from headache and without evidence of primary structural abnormality.

The word "migraine" is French and derives from the Greek *hemicrania*, meaning that the pain involves only half the head at one time. This is usually the case, but about one-third of headaches with all the other characteristics of migraine affect both sides of the head at the same time. What are these other characteristics? The most common are nausea, vomiting, and sensitivity to light (photophobia). The problem in defining migraine is that the nature of the attack varies from patient to patient and may even change from one headache to another in the same person.

The Natural History of Migraine

Migrainous symptoms may first appear in early childhood and alter in character as the child grows. A child may suffer from vomiting and abdominal pain (bilious attacks) at an early age whenever there is a party or some other excitement. A little later, the child may complain of headache accompanying the vomiting attacks, which recur every few months. At puberty, the episodes may be heralded by shimmering or blurred eyesight or even by spectacular zigzags of color that move slowly across the field of vision, leaving blank spots behind where vision is impaired or completely lost (see Figure 4.1). The headaches have a 60 percent chance of disappearing in the late teens but may persist, in which case nausea is often less prominent and vomiting may cease to be part of the attack (14). Those children who do lose their headaches in adolescence have about a 30 percent chance of recurrence in later years, so that about 60 percent of migrainous children will still be subject to migraine in their thirties. In middle life, the headaches may cease and the patient may be left with the visual disturbance only, which is then called a migraine equivalent. There are no inviolable rules to the game. Migraine equivalents may appear early in life and the other symptoms may be added later on. Some people have milder headaches between the more severe attacks, which makes it difficult to decide where migraine ends and tension headache begins. Some develop migraine for the first time in their fifties, but it is more common for the migrainous tendency to abate gradually. Affected adults have a 70 percent chance of losing their headaches or improving substantially over the course of fifteen years or so. Let us look at all variations on the theme of migraine, bearing in mind that a patient may slide from one category into another on different occasions.

Classification of Migraine

Migraine is most easily classified by the presence or absence of neurological symptoms, such as distorted vision (ripples, flashes of light, or zigzags in front of the eyes), weakness of one side of the body, a pins-and-needles sensation around the mouth or on one or both sides of the body, or difficulty in choosing words (see Figure 4.2). If such symptoms precede or

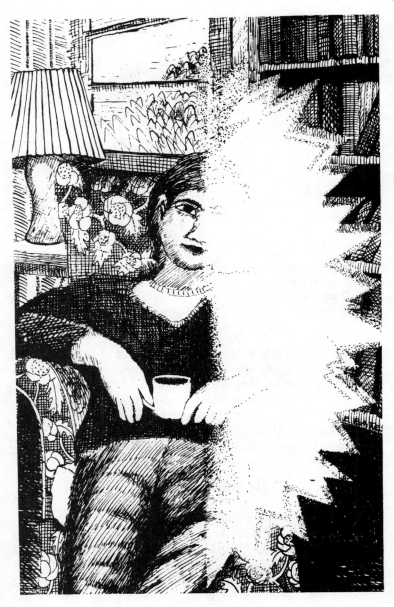

4.1 *Visual disturbance in classical migraine. A semicircular zigzag pattern moves across the field of vision, leaving blank patches be-hind. Drawn by Edwina Bates.*

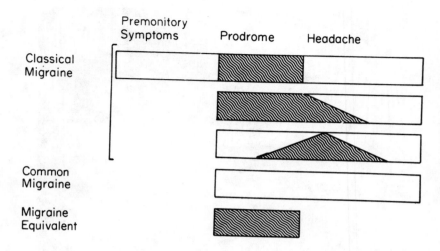

4.2 *Types of migraine. In classical migraine the headache is preceded or accompanied by neurological symptoms (crosshatched areas), unlike common migraine. If neurological symptoms occur on their own, the episode is called a migraine equivalent.*

accompany migraine headache, the condition is called classical migraine. If such symptoms appear on their own without any headache following, they are known as migraine equivalents. If neurological symptoms persist for more than twenty-four hours after the headache ceases, the condition is classified as complicated migraine. If there are no neurological symptoms at all, the headaches are termed common migraine.

Early Warning Symptoms

Whether migraine is of the classical or common variety, about 20 percent of patients experience premonitory symptoms for up to twenty-four hours before the attacks start (Figure 4.2). These include changes in mood, changes in appetite, and drowsiness. People may feel elated, on top of the world, and full of energy. They can fly through the day's work and accomplish twice as much as usual. The canny ones among them may recognize that this heralds a migraine headache the following day. Occasionally the mood change can be just the opposite, so that they feel depressed and irritable.

Victims may feel intense hunger or a craving for sweet things and may consume a whole box of cookies or chocolates. When headache follows the next day, they may blame the headache on eating chocolate, whereas their chocolate consumption was only signaling the approach of migraine. Some may feel drowsy before a migraine headache and may yawn incessantly. All these warning symptoms arise in a deep-seated part of the brain, the hypothalamus.

Classical Migraine

Visual hallucinations form part of the migraine in about one-third of migrainous patients, commonly appearing before the headache as a prodome or aura lasting for twenty to forty-five minutes (Figure 4.2). These may take the form of a semi-circle of angled lines, white or colored, that jitter to and fro, slowly moving across the field of vision and leaving blank spots behind (Figure 4.1). These were named fortification spectra by Dr. John Fothergill, a London physician, who wrote in 1788: "After breakfast, if much toast and butter has been used it begins with a singular kind of glimmering in the sight; objects swiftly change their apparent position, surrounded with luminous angles like those of a fortification. Giddiness then comes on with headache and sickness" (73).

While only 10 percent of patients experience fortification spectra, some 25 percent see unformed flashes of light or color associated with a patchy impairment of vision that may obliterate the right or left half of any objects viewed. Sometimes the whole field of vision may close in, leaving only the central part (tunnel vision). Edward Liveing (1873) quoted a poetic description from one of his patients who saw "sparks or bright beads in incessant motion" that reminded him of "the effects produced by the rapid gyrations of the lesser water beetles as I have seen them in patches on rivers and ponds in the bright sunshine" (73).

"Pins and needles" are felt in the face or limbs by one-third of patients, and about 4 percent may develop weakness on one side of the body resembling a stroke. They may also find it difficult to understand conversation or select the right word to describe their thoughts. The symptoms usually clear up within the space of an hour as the headache develops. The headache itself is indistinguishable from common migraine.

Common Migraine

Common migraine is a recurrent headache of at least moderate severity that is usually associated with nausea and hypersensitivity to light, sounds, or smells. It affects only one side of the head in about two-thirds of patients and commonly starts as a dull ache in the back of the head and upper neck or in one temple. It may extend to become a bar of pain between the forehead and neck (Figure 1.1) or spread over the whole of that side of the head. It may even cover one half of the face, involving the nostril, cheek, and jaw. This is called lower-half headache or facial migraine.

During migraine headache, light may become dazzling or even give rise to pain (photophobia). Some 80 percent of patients find light unpleasant and prefer to lie in a darkened room. Pope used the old English word *megrim* for migraine in the following allusion to photophobia:

> *And screen'd in shades from day's detested glare,*
> *She sighs for ever on her pensive bed,*
> *Pain at her side, and megrim at her head.*
>   Alexander Pope, "Rape of the Lock," Canto 4

Sensory perceptions may also be heightened. For some patients, sounds appear unnaturally loud and smells more intense during the headache phase. The scalp may be very sensitive to touch, so that sufferers cannot bear to brush their hair or lie on the affected side. Muscles of the head and neck feel tender. All these symptoms suggest that some damping-down mechanism within the central nervous system has been released, reducing restriction on the inflow of sensations.

Nausea may precede the headache but commonly develops with it. In about half the patients with common or classical migraine, this culminates in vomiting on at least some occasions. Some 16 percent of people notice diarrhea at the same time.

Patients usually look pale and their eyes appear dark and sunken, although occasionally an individual may flush with the attack. In about one-third of patients, the arteries may pulsate excessively in the temples, and veins will stand out on the forehead, in which case pressure over the distended vessels usually eases the pain. Some people retain fluid with migraine, causing their faces to appear swollen.

The headache may last for only a few hours but more commonly persists until the patient goes to sleep. The person may awaken feeling washed out with no more than a dull ache and a sensitive scalp as a souvenir of the previously severe pain. It is rare, but not unheard of, for a headache to persist for days.

Other Varieties of Migraine

Basilar Artery Migraine (with Loss of Balance and Fainting)

In 1961, Dr. Edwin Bickerstaff of the University of Birmingham described a form of migraine that was particularly common in adolescents (12). Along with the visual disturbances of classical migraine, these young patients developed giddiness, loss of balance, and slurred speech, followed by aching mainly in the back of the head. About one-third fainted at the height of the attack. These symptoms all pointed to a disturbance of the hind brain, the brain stem and cerebellum (the center that maintains the sense of balance). The one connecting link that could explain why all these symptoms occurred together was the role played by the basilar artery, which runs along the base of the brain, supplying the brain stem and cerebellum with blood and then branching to course backward to the visual cortex (see Figure 4.3). Bickerstaff suggested that a spasm of the artery or its branches deprived these parts of the brain of blood and caused this sequence of symptoms. Minor symptoms of basilar artery migraine are quite common, for about a quarter of all patients notice giddiness, faintness, and slurred speech on some occasions. At the other end of the spectrum, severe attacks can lead to epileptic fits and temporary loss of memory.

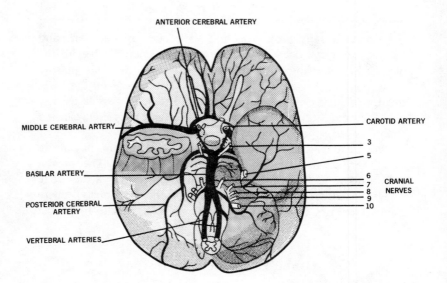

ANTERIOR CEREBRAL ARTERY

MIDDLE CEREBRAL ARTERY

BASILAR ARTERY

POSTERIOR CEREBRAL ARTERY

VERTEBRAL ARTERIES

CAROTID ARTERY

3
5
6
7
8
9
10

CRANIAL NERVES

4.3 *The base of the brain, showing the main blood vessels and cranial nerves. The two vertebral arteries unite to form the basilar artery. The basilar artery gives rise to the posterior cerebral arteries, which supply the visual cortex at the back of the brain. Basilar artery migraine thus affects vision as well as balance and consciousness. The cranial nerves are numbered, with 5 designating the trigeminal nerve, 9 the glossopharyngeal, and 10 the vagus. Blood vessels may compress these nerves to cause neuralgia (see chapter 10).*

Confusional States and Stupor

In migraine, the reduction in blood flow to the brain can make people confused and irrational. Concentration is impaired, and victims may make simple errors in speech and writing (see Figure 4.4). One left her baby in the bath and was found walking aimlessly down the street outside her house. Others may become agitated and aggressive. A mild, accidental blow to the head can induce confusional attacks in some children (47). Falling off a chair, banging heads together, or any slight knock or jar can cause a susceptible child to become irrational for minutes or even hours. Confusion may be associated with blurring or loss of vision and is usually followed by

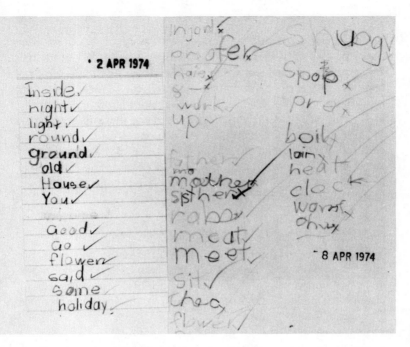

4.4 *Confusional states in migraine. A child's usually neat and correct handwriting and spelling (left) deteriorated with the onset of migraine headache (right).*

headache. Such attacks are very frightening and may suggest concussion or other forms of brain damage. However, they are often the initial manifestation of migraine, in which case, with repeated attacks, the diagnosis becomes clear. Rarely, sufferers become unconscious with migraine headache and can be roused only with difficulty, a condition known as migraine stupor, which may continue for hours or even days (71).

Hemiplegic Migraine
(with Weakness on One Side of the Body)

This form of migraine resembles a stroke and may progress until the arm and leg on the same side are completely paralyzed. Paralysis usually lasts for a few hours and then clears up, although some patients may be left with residual weakness after repeated attacks. Hemiplegic migraine usually is hereditary. Patients are advised not to smoke cigarettes or to take contraceptive pills, as the combination increases the tendency for clots to form in the blood vessels. As the blood flow to the brain is severely reduced in hemiplegic migraine, there is a real risk of clot formation leading to permanent stroke. Sometimes children have attacks in which the weakness affects different sides of the body on different occasions (alternating hemiplegia of childhood), and the connection with migraine may not be immediately apparent.

Ophthalmoplegic Migraine (with Double Vision)

Ophthalmoplegia means paralysis of one or more of the muscles moving the eyes. When this happens, the eyes move out of alignment and the person sees double. Minor degrees of visual disturbance are quite common in migraine, but sometimes there is an obvious squint.

Retinal Migraine (with Loss of Vision in One Eye)

Infrequently, the vessels in the retina of one eye may go into spasm, causing dimness or loss of vision in the eye. This is quite different from the more common visual problem in migraine, which involves the left or the right half of the field of vision (Figures 4.1, 6.3), because the seeing part of the brain is affected. In retinal migraine the eye itself is involved, so that the sufferer loses sight in the affected eye but can see normally from the other. The sight gradually clears, leaving an ache behind the eye or a generalized headache.

Abdominal Migraine (Recurrent Stomach Pains in Childhood)

About 20 percent of migrainous children have periodic abdominal pains, compared with about 4 percent of children who do not suffer from headache. A past history of childhood vomiting attacks is given by about one-quarter of patients with migraine. Abdominal pains and vomiting may be part of the migraine attack, and it is probable that they can occur on their own as a recurrent migraine equivalent.

How Common Is Migraine?

The estimated prevalence of migraine varies according to the criteria used for diagnosis. A survey of almost 15,000 people conducted by the British Migraine Trust in 1975 found that 10 percent of males and 16 percent of females suffered from one-sided headaches with migrainous characteristics (46). A survey in Denmark reported that migraine became progressively more common as children got older, increasing from about 3 percent at the age of seven years to 9 percent at the age of fifteen (27). After puberty, the prevalence of migraine in women increased to 19 percent during the reproductive years of life but leveled out at about 11 percent in men.

Women are affected by migraine more often than men, with the ratio varying from 3:2 to 3:1 in various surveys.

Conclusions

From the descriptions of the many varieties of migraine, it can be seen that migraine is not simply a severe headache. It would be naive to expect that one explanation necessarily applies to all types of migraine and that one cure will be found. We now know why forms of migraine differ (see chapter 6) and can indeed keep most migraine cases under control (see chapter 7), even if we cannot offer a permanent cure. Before we go into these questions, it would be a good idea to consider the sort of people who get migraine, the frequency of migraine attacks, and certain life events that may precipitate headaches in susceptible people (see chapter 5).

5

CLINICAL FEATURES OF MIGRAINE

The Family Tendency to Migraine

Migraine usually runs in families. A close family member is affected by migraine in 60 percent of sufferers, compared with only 16 percent of the general population. It appears that the pain-control system and the related neurotransmitters are different in migrainous subjects, being more sensitive to changes in the body itself or in the outside world. The body is regulated by internal clocks, so that changes take place each day, week, or month at about the same time; some headaches are brought on by these changes. Other headaches are precipitated by some external change, and avoiding such trigger factors can reduce the frequency of headache. Thus, any sudden change in the internal or external environment can upset the delicate balance of the nervous system and cause migraine headaches in those with a hereditary susceptibility to migraine. Let us see whether there is a typical migraine personality and then examine those factors that can switch migraine headaches on and off.

Personality and Intelligence

In the past, migraine patients have received some consolation from the assurance that the disorder strikes only those who are intelligent and sensitive. While the second part of this proposition may be true, the evidence unfortunately does not support the idea that migraine sufferers are brighter than average. Professor B. Bille, University Hospital, Uppsala, Sweden, did not find any difference in the grades achieved by migrainous and nonmigrainous groups of children, and he could not detect any indications of greater ambition in the migrainous children (13).

The person susceptible to migraine is said to be tense, meticulous, and obsessional by nature (see Figure 5.1). In a group of five hundred patients studied by Dr. George Selby and myself at the Northcott Neurological Centre, Sydney, 23 percent were found to be unduly tidy and house-proud and had the habit of double-checking their actions (100). Another 22 percent were overactive, restless, and tense individuals who found it very difficult to relax. Definite symptoms of anxiety were present in another 13 percent who experienced difficulty in sleeping, tremor of the hands, a tendency to take deep, sighing breaths, and feelings of depression.

To come to any valid conclusions, it is necessary to compare a control group of similar age, sex, and social background who are not subject to migraine. Professor Bille found that mi-

SEPTEMBER							1	2	3		5	6	7	8	9		11	12	13	14	15	16	17	18	19	20	21	22	23	24 25 26 27 28 29 30
OCTOBER		3	4	5	6	7	8	9	10	11	12	13	14	15	16	17	18	19	20	21	22	23	24	25	26	27	28	29	30	31
NOVEMBER			1	2	3			6	7	8	9	10	11		14	15	16	17	18			20	21	22		24	25	26	27	28	29 30
DECEMBER				1	2	3	4	5	6	7	8	9	10	11	12	13	14	15	16	17		19	20	21	22	23	24	25	26	27 28 29
JANUARY	1	2	3	4	5					11	12	13	14	15	16			19	20	21	22	23		25	26	27	28	29	30	31
FEBRUARY			1	2	3		5	6	7	8	9	10	11	12	13	14	15	16	17	18	19		21	22	23		26	27	28
MARCH		1	2	3	4	5	6	7	8	9	10	11	12	13	14	15	16		18	19	20	21	22	23	24	25	26	27	28	29	31
APRIL	1	2	3	4	5	6	7	8	9		11								20	21	22	23	24	25		27	28	29	30
MAY		2	3	4	5		7		10	11	12	13	14	15	16	17	18	19	20	21		23	24	25	26	27	28	29	30	31
JUNE			2	3	4	5	6	7	8	9	10	11	12	13	14	15	16	17	18	19	20		22	23	24	25	26		28	29 30 31
JULY	1		3	4	5	6	7	8		10	11	12	13	14	15	16		18	19	20	21	22	23	24		26	27	28	29	30	31
AUGUST		1	2	3	4	5	6	7	8	9	10	11	12	13	14	15	16	17		19	20	21	22	23	24	25	26	27	28	29 30 31
SEPTEMBER							7	8	9																					

WEEKEND	PUBLIC HOL.	HOLIDAY	OVERTIME	MIGRAINE	SPECIAL

5.1 *A record of headaches and precipitating factors kept by a meticulous migrainous patient.*

grainous children were significantly more anxious, tense, sensitive, and vulnerable to frustration than the control children.
In addition, the migraine-prone children were more tidy and
physically weaker than their peers. Dr. Rita Henryk-Gutt and
Dr. W. Linford Rees of St. Bartholomew's Hospital, London,
studied fifty men and fifty women from the Civil Service (51).
They compared them with matched controls, who suffered
from other forms of headache, and with another group who
were not prone to any kind of headache. They found that
migraine sufferers had not been exposed to more stress than
the other groups but that they had a stronger reaction to all
forms of stress. They could not confirm previous suggestions
that the migraine victims were more obsessional or ambitious.
More than half the episodes of migraine were attributed to some
obviously stressful event.

Recent studies using standard psychological tests have not
demonstrated any definite deviation from normalcy in migrainous patients, nor have they confirmed the traditional view of the
perfectionist, rigid nature of migraine sufferers. Yet we can still
see these tendencies in some patients (Figure 5.1). To general-
ize, the typical migraine personality is normal, but perhaps a
bit on the sensitive side.

Internal Clocks

Some patients are prone to a headache once each month,
which for women may occur at the time of their menstrual
periods. Others have a headache once a week, often on the
same day each week, even if there is no obvious stress attached
to that day's events. An unfortunate few are prone to daily
headaches, which may awaken them from sleep in the early
hours of the morning. Cyclical events in the body are determined by biological clocks, nerve centers in the brain that
generate rhythmic activity. Some of these promote the release
of hormones into the bloodstream to carry out tasks in different
parts of the body. For example, the secretion of female hormones, ovulation, and changes in the lining of the uterus are
under the control of chemical messengers sent from the brain.

The prime example of an internal clock is the small area of gray matter perched above the optic nerves that carries information from the eye. Because it is situated over the crossing of the optic nerve fibers (the chiasm) it is called the suprachiasmatic nucleus. It receives fibers from the optic nerve that signal whether it is day or night outside. This information sets the nucleus on a twenty-four-hour cycle so that we feel sleepy at an appropriate time and wake up in the morning. During the night there are different phases of deep and light sleep that change every ninety minutes or so. The onset of a migraine headache will often occur after one of these transition periods. However, sleeping often gets rid of migraine headache, and many patients with headache try to sleep for this reason.

Even if we avoid external trigger factors, we cannot escape our internal clocks, which can switch on migraine at predetermined intervals like an unwanted alarm bell. Dr. Arnold Friedman, formerly affiliated with Montefiore Hospital in New York, told of one patient who has an occupation that takes him through the world from the Himalayas in Tibet to Somaliland, indeed from the highest altitudes to the lowest, from the wettest to the driest regions—experiencing climatic, food, and cultural changes. But his migraine remains, for he carries his personal environment with him (40).

Trigger Factors

Many people can identify specific circumstances that bring on migraine headache. These are not necessarily *causes* of migraine but may set in motion the machinery that results in an attack. The most direct of these triggers is a blow to the head.

Blows to the Head ("Football Player's Migraine")

Professor W. B. Matthews of Oxford University described a group of young men who developed blurred vision within two minutes after being hit on the head by a football or punched in a boxing match (77). The visual disturbance was followed by typical migraine headache with vomiting. Curiously enough, none was subject to headache on other occasions. Members of an American University Team experienced flashing lights in front of their eyes, blurred vision, "pins and needles" in the limbs, and loss of memory after a comparatively minor blow to the head, not always followed by headache (10). Similar instances have occurred among schoolboys playing rugby football. Children are particularly liable to develop symptoms of classical migraine after a slight blow to the head, as noted in chapter 4 in the discussion on confusional states (47). It is not known whether the injury acts on the brain stem or directly jars the blood vessels of the brain to reduce blood flow and cause these migrainous symptoms.

Pressure on the Head ("Goggle Migraine")

A thirty-six-year-old neurologist wrote to the *New England Journal of Medicine* in 1983 and described throbbing headaches in both temples coming on one to two hours after swim training (90). Some headaches were preceded by typical scintillations of vision and one by the loss of one-half of the field of vision. They ceased when he stopped using tight swim goggles and recurred when he started to wear them again. He eventually found that the solution was to wear goggles with a single soft-rubber rim that fitted around both eyes and did not require a tight head-strap.

Changes in Barometric Pressure

Classical migraine has been reported by airplane crews flying at a high altitude and, more commonly, occurring five to thirty minutes after descent. It has also been reported after recovery from simulated altitudes of thirty to thirty-eight thousand feet in a low-pressure chamber (39). It tends to occur repeatedly in certain individuals, particularly those who have previously suffered from migraine, and not at all in others. Headache is also a common symptom of "acute mountain sickness" when healthy people remain at a simulated altitude of fourteen to fifteen thousand feet for several hours (57). It is caused by swelling of the scalp arteries and is relieved by applying pressure on these vessels or by prescribed drugs that cause the arteries to constrict.

Decompression after simulated diving to depths of 66 to 135 feet below sea level in a high-pressure (hyperbaric) chamber has also been known to precipitate migraine (4). Four out of thirty individuals who were exposed weekly to such pressure changes experienced the sensation of flashing lights, "heat waves," or rainbows in front of their eyes, with blurring of vision ten to ninety minutes after decompression, in most cases followed by headache. The visual disturbances disappeared promptly with oxygen therapy, but the headache still followed in three out of four subjects. All four were subject to migraine at other times, but the induced attacks differed from the spontaneous attacks, being milder in some and more severe in others.

The arteries of the scalp and brain appear to be very sensitive to the pressure of oxygen in the blood and particularly to any sudden change in oxygen level.

Weather

Many patients believe that sudden changes in the weather, particularly thunderstorms, may be responsible for migraine. Although the drop in barometric pressure is not nearly as dramatic as that in compression chambers, the possibility that it plays some part in triggering migraine, perhaps by increasing nervous tension, cannot be denied. Professor F. G. Sulman and his colleagues at the Hebrew University, Jerusalem, have studied the effect of a hot, dry wind, known as the Sharav, in Israel (106, 107). They point out that cool winds like the French Mistral or Canadian Chinook do not usually cause headache but that "hot winds of ill repute" are notorious for causing irritability, depression, and headache. They list the Santa Ana of southern California, Arizona desert winds, the Argentine Zonda, the Sirocco of the Mediterranean, the Maltese Xlokk, the Chamsin of Arab countries, the Sharav of the Old Testament, the Foehn of Switzerland, southern Germany, and Austria, and the North Winds of Melbourne. They found that a weather front with increased ionization of the air (electrical charges that may cause lightning) arrived one to two days before the hot, dry wind, and believed that this might be responsible for the symptoms. Of two hundred patients who developed symptoms simultaneous with the arrival of the Sharav, eighty excreted excessive amounts of serotonin (a substance thought to play a part in causing migraine). Migraine was prevented in seventy of these cases by the use of pizotifen (Sandomigran), a drug that counteracted the effect of serotonin. At present, this prescription drug is not available in the United States.

Less dramatic changes in weather do not appear to have much effect on the tendency to migraine. Dr. R. E. Cull of the Royal Infirmary, Edinburgh, correlated the incidence of migraine with changes in the barometric pressure on the day of headache and for the preceding forty-eight hours (25). Curiously, the mean barometric pressure was higher on migraine days than on headache-free days, but an increase in barometric pressure of more than fifteen millibars over the preceding twenty-four hours heralded a day of relative freedom. Cull concluded that the minor changes in attack rate could be explained by indirect factors such as the lack of glare on cool, cloudy days.

Stress (Emotions, Glare, Noise)

Some degree of stress must be associated with receiving a blow on the head or being locked in a decompression chamber. One patient of mine regularly had a migraine headache the day after he had his hair cut. It would be an exaggeration to classify a haircut as a head injury, Samson notwithstanding, Perhaps this may be regarded as a form of stress. Emotional stress can certainly provoke a migraine headache. Several of my patients have mentioned that the distortion of vision that heralds an attack started within minutes of an emotional shock. In their survey of migraine patients, Dr. Henryk-Gutt and Dr. Rees found that about half their patients attributed the onset of attacks to some obviously stressful event (51).

Other factors such as noise, glare, odors, or unpleasant weather conditions, like hot, dry winds, can induce nervous tension and promote an attack of migraine. Some 50 percent of patients attribute their headaches either to the glare that results from driving a car into the sun or the eyestrain from watching movies or television. Sensitivity to noise was described by the French physician Antoine Labarraque in 1837 in the following terms (73):

> We all know that it is not everyone who can, with impunity, do himself the pleasure of assisting at certain theatrical representations where the glory of France is daily celebrated with noise and smoke. And how many good citizens are there not, tried patriots, whom the threatening of a migraine, infallibly brought on by the unaccustomed din of drums and military music, forcibly hinders from taking part in our civic fêtes, and joining their companies on grand review days.

Relaxation After Stress (Weekend Headache)

When headaches appear only on weekends, there is no need necessarily to blame the domestic situation. It is probable that during prolonged periods of stress, the scalp vessels are constricted by the nervous system or by chemicals in the bloodstream such as serotonin and norepinephrine. When the working week ends and the subject is at last able to relax, the vessels tend to dilate and cause migraine headache. Dr. Arnold P. Friedman, in his essay "The Headache in History, Literature and Legend," quotes from a letter by Sigmund Freud, who wrote, "My health has been excellent—regulated by a slight migraine on Sundays" (41). Sleeping in on Saturday or Sunday mornings may also be a factor causing weekend headache, possibly by disturbing the internal clock that normally regulates sleeping and waking.

Just as relaxation may induce headache, a sudden change in emotion may cure it. Dr. Friedman also quotes an example of this. Ulysses S. Grant, general of the Union armies in the Civil War, was "suffering very severely from a sick headache" and spent the night bathing his feet in hot water and mustard and putting mustard plasters on his wrists and neck. The next day he received a letter from Robert E. Lee, the Confederate general, announcing that he was willing to surrender. Grant wrote in his journal, "I was still suffering from the sick headache: but the instant I saw the contents of the note I was cured." He later commented, "The pain in my head seemed to leave me the moment I got Lee's letter." Antoine Labarraque described the prevention of an attack by a sudden shock. A thirty-five-year-old woman suffered from migraine every eight to ten days. "One day when she felt an attack coming on, going to look at her face in the glass, her cap caught fire and burnt her forehead. The expected seizure never came on, and furthermore, she had no return for some years."

Sleep

A jailer in Shakespeare's *Cymbeline* says, "Indeed, sir, he that sleeps feels not the toothache." Unfortunately, sir and madame, he that sleeps does feel the headache. Indeed it is not uncommon for someone to be awakened by a headache in the small hours of the morning, or for one to be present when the person awakens at the usual time. Dr. J. D. Dexter and Dr. E. D. Weitzman of Montefiore Hospital in New York studied a number of patients who were plagued with nocturnal headache by recording their brain waves, the electrical activity of the brain, while they slept (28). This was done by attaching electrodes to the scalp, and the changes in electrical activity were written out as an electroencephalogram (EEG). It is well known that the EEG pattern alters during the various stages of sleep. At intervals throughout the night, sleep lightens. As this happens, the brain waves indicate partial arousal and the eyes move from side to side. This is known as the rapid eye movement (REM) phase of sleep. At the onset of REM sleep, all sorts of things may happen, such as dreams, nocturnal emissions, and even bed-wetting. All the nocturnal headaches observed were related to the REM phase of sleep. It is interesting to note that dreams and headache may become intermingled. Edward Liveing quoted an example: "Dr. Airy says his attacks sometimes occur in the night, and that he has had an indistinct consciousness of having experienced the visual phenomena in his sleep, mixed up with his dreams, and he awakes in the second, or headache stage." When the cycle of sleeping and waking is altered in phase (for example, by air travel), headaches also change in timing, but maintain their relation to the REM phase of sleep. Whether REM sleep and its associated headache is related to changes in brain chemistry, to the accumulation of carbon dioxide in the bloodstream, or to other factors is at present unknown.

Foods

Headaches have long been attributed to digestive disturbances and to the flow of bile, one of the digestive juices. The vomiting attacks of childhood, often migrainous in origin, are still referred to as "bilious attacks." The Roman physician Galen commented almost two thousand years ago, "How constantly do we see the head attacked with pain when yellow bile is contained in the stomach: as also the pain forthwith ceasing when the bile has been vomited."

The belief that migraine may be triggered by eating certain kinds of foods is of equally long standing. Dr. Fothergill wrote in 1778: "It is most clear that the headache proceeds from the stomach, not the reverse" (73). He blamed certain foods, particularly "melted butter, fat meats, spices, meat pies, hot buttered toast, and malt liquors when strong and hoppy." Fothergill went on, "From many incontestible proofs that butter in considerable quantity is injurious, it is less used in many families. Nothing more speedily and effectively gives the sick-headache, and sometimes within a few hours."

When Dr. George Selby and I analyzed the case histories of five hundred migraine patients, we found that 25 percent attributed the onset to eating certain foods (compared with 67 percent who blamed emotional disturbances and 47 percent who mentioned glare). Fats, fried foods, chocolate, and oranges were most often cited, but tomatoes, pineapples, and onions were also occasionally mentioned (100). Before we get carried away with the food-sensitivity hypothesis, we should consider some experiments using placebos carried out by the late Harold G. Wolff at New York Hospital (114). "With the administration of chocolate disguised in capsules for those allegedly sensitive to chocolate, or milk given through a stomach tube to those who were said to be sensitive to milk, the results did not confirm the earlier work. No headache ensued." A study from the London Hospital of twenty-five patients who claimed that their headaches were invariably brought on by eating chocolate or any cocoa products could not find any relationship (83). In eighty trials, only thirteen headaches followed the taking of chocolate, while eight came on after eating a substance that had been made to look like chocolate.

In our own clinic, thirty-four migrainous patients were skin-tested for food and other allergies. Twenty-three patients who gave positive reactions avoided the appropriate allergens for several months without reduction in the frequency of attacks. Ten patients were placed on low-fat diets for up to six months, but again the pattern of attacks remained unaltered.

Cheese has been cited as a factor. Dr. Edda Hanington and her colleagues at the Wellcome Trust in London found that tyramine, which is present in cheese, could produce a migraine headache in susceptible patients, whereas lactose given in identical capsules rarely did (48). However, another group in London repeated this experiment and found that there was no more incidence of headache after ingesting the same amount of tyramine than there was after ingesting the inactive substance with which tyramine was compared (82).

Two studies carried out in London in 1980 and 1983 have claimed success in reducing the frequency of migraine headache by eliminating offending foods from the diet, but other trials have been unsuccessful (84, 35). If patients are convinced that certain foods precipitate attacks, these foods should obviously be avoided, but there is no need for everyone who is subject to migraine to eliminate chocolate, cheese, or oranges from his diet.

Missing Meals

While it is doubtful that foods trigger migraine, there is little question that missing meals may cause headache in some people, probably by lowering the blood sugar level. Dr. J. N. Blau and Professor J. N. Cumings of the National Hospital for Nervous Diseases in London found that six out of twelve migrainous subjects who did not eat for nineteen hours developed a migraine headache (15). A follow-up of this study by Dr. Blau and Dr. D. A. Pyke involved the investigation of thirty-six patients with both migraine and diabetes (16). Six patients noted that missing a meal provoked migraine headache, and another four were subject to headaches at night, when their blood sugar fell as a result of insulin treatment. The patients could differentiate between the onset of migraine and the generalized headache that usually accompanied a severe drop in the blood sugar level after insulin, and some felt that they could prevent the development of migraine by eating as soon as they felt the first symptoms. The effect of lowering blood sugar by giving insulin to nondiabetic migraine patients is less effective. Dr. John Pearce of Hull Royal Infirmary, Hull, England, found that only two out of twenty responded with a headache (89).

Alcohol

Wine was mentioned as a precipitant of migraine in the days of the Roman Empire. Cornelius Celsus, a friend of the emperor Tiberius, wrote in about 30 A.D. of a headache "sometimes afflicting the whole head, at other times a part of it," contracted by drinking wine and recurring throughout life (24). Edward Liveing in 1873 commented, "Some few individuals cannot tolerate any kind of beer or wine" (73). He quoted a case: "One gentleman, a most intelligent member of our profession . . . told me that for twenty years or more he could never take the smallest quantity of wine (and he mentioned the sacramental wine as an instance) . . . without infallibly producing a headache." In general, Liveing considered "wine, especially if taken in large quantity, or of a different quality from that to which the patient is accustomed, or if several kinds are taken, will often occasion an attack; but this is not the case when the same kind is taken daily with moderation and regularity; and with many patients it is very beneficial." In fact, he states that "a full dose of Brandy or other alcoholic stimulant, if taken sufficiently early, will occasionally disperse an incipient seizure [of migraine]."

I have not encountered any patient who could prevent an attack by taking alcohol in any form. In fact, it is usually a useful way to distinguish a vascular headache, such as migraine, from tension headache. Tension headache is often relieved by alcohol; vascular headaches are almost invariably made worse. The reason for this is that alcohol is a dilator of blood vessels and that the pain of migraine arises from vessels that are already dilated.

I have seen many patients, including neurologists and other physicians, who are convinced that their migraines follow the drinking of red wines, but who may enjoy white wines without any problem. One interesting point is that a trigger such as red wine may not be effective immediately after a spontaneous headache or for some days afterward until the vessels regain their sensitivity. It is as though the vessels are exhausted after an attack and enter a refractory period during which they will not respond, however great the provocation.

Exercise

A number of patients develop migraine after extreme exertion, like playing a hard game of tennis. This is discussed in chapter 3 under the heading "Exertional Vascular Headaches." Such headaches can usually be prevented by taking suitable medication, such as ergotamine tartrate or indomethacin, before the exercise starts. These medications prevent painful swelling of the scalp arteries.

Hormonal Changes

The character of migraine frequently undergoes a transformation at puberty. The more dramatic symptoms of visual and sensory disturbance often appear then for the first time, and the headaches may become more intense than ever before. In pubescent girls, the incidence of migraine increases until twice as many girls are affected as boys. In some 60 percent of female patients, headaches occur before or during menstruation. In the last six months of pregnancy, the majority obtain some relief, only to have the headache attacks recur shortly after the delivery of their baby. Dr. Michael Anthony and I studied 120 women who had undergone 252 pregnancies and found that relief during pregnancy was more common in those women whose migraine had previously been associated with their menstrual periods (64 percent) than in those in whom it had not (48 percent) (64). A few women notice the onset of migraine for the first time during pregnancy, but these are in the minority.

Dr. Brian Somerville in my department at the Prince Henry Hospital, Sydney, studied levels of female hormones in the blood throughout the menstrual cycle in a number of migrainous women (104, 105). The headache always started while the levels of estrogen and progesterone were falling before the onset of menstruation. Somerville found that injecting progesterone to maintain a high level in the blood did not prevent the onset of migraine, but that injecting estrogen would delay the headache until the level in the blood finally dropped. We may conclude that the fall of the level of estrogen in some way triggers the onset of migraine.

Menstruation occurs when the constriction of the small blood vessels that supply the soft inner lining of the uterus cause the superficial layers to slough off and discharge in the menstrual flow. There is some evidence that members of a group of substances called the prostaglandins are responsible for this constriction of vessels in the uterus, and it is also known that other members of this group can cause migraine if injected into the bloodstream of people who have never had a migraine attack before. It is tempting to guess that the lowering of the female hormone estradiol in the blood releases prostaglandins. These may set in motion the vascular changes of menstruation and, as a side effect in some unfortunate individuals, the vascular changes that result in migraine.

Oral contraceptives contain different combinations of synthetic estrogens and progesterones that prevent ovulation. They do not really simulate the changes of pregnancy, because the blood level is permitted to fall away at monthly intervals to allow menstruation to take place. A few patients notice an improvement in their migraine when they start taking one form or other of "the pill," but in most patients the frequency and intensity of headaches increase, and some notice additional minor vascular headaches. Almost all patients continue to have a migraine attack before their periods. Those whose migraine is intensified by oral contraceptives must decide whether to continue taking them, which would mean adding daily medication to diminish their sensitivity to migraine (like driving a car with the accelerator and the brake being applied together). Alternatively, they can stop the pill and choose another contraceptive method. When patients have severe intracranial symptoms with their attacks—speech difficulty, pins and needles, weakness down one side of the body, or loss of vision—our clinic strongly advises that they stop taking oral contraceptives. In a number of instances, sufferers from this form of migraine have sustained a permanent disability resembling a stroke when they have continued to take the pill regularly. In ordinary forms of migraine, common migraine, the choice is left to the patient.

Epilepsy and Allergy

An analogy has often been drawn between epilepsy and migraine, because both often appear suddenly in those who are otherwise well, and both may recur at fairly regular intervals. To assess whether epilepsy was more common in migraine subjects, Dr. Michael Anthony and I compared a group of five hundred patients who were subject to typical migraine attacks with one hundred patients who had only tension headaches (64). There was no difference between the two groups in their liability to epilepsy or in any family history of epilepsy. Professor Bille came to identical conclusions in his study of migrainous children (13).

A similar analysis has been made of adults and children to see whether allergic disorders (asthma, hay fever, hives, and eczema) were more common in patients who suffered from migraine. The frequency of allergy was found to be no greater than that in the populations with which they were compared (64). This does not mean that an allergic attack may not occasionally trigger migraine or that a severe migraine headache may not occasionally precipitate an epileptic attack in someone *who is already predisposed to epilepsy from some other cause.* This is a different matter from trying to link these disorders to a common underlying mechanism, for which there is no evidence at present.

Age of Onset

On two separate occasions I have analyzed the characteristics of five hundred patients attending a neurological clinic. Women comprised 60 percent of the patients in the first series of five hundred, reported with Dr. George Selby, and 75 percent of the second, reported with Dr. Michael Anthony (100, 64). In each series the initial attack of migraine was experienced at ten years of age or younger (see Figures 5.2a, 8.1). The youngest subject I can recall was a baby of three months whose mother remembered episodes in which he cried, held his head, and vomited. When he was old enough to describe the accompanying headache, it became clear that these episodes had all the hallmarks of migraine. The onset of migraine at fifty years of age or older is rare, but migraine equivalents may appear in the later years of life. This often gives rise to concern about the possibility of an impending stroke, but such fears appear to be unwarranted.

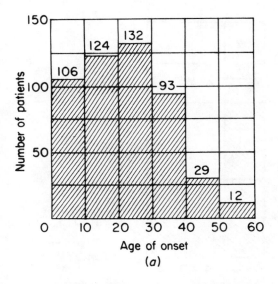

(a)

5.2 *Data gathered from 500 migrainous patients. The age at which headaches started is shown in (a).*

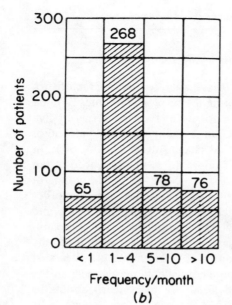

The frequency of attacks occurring each month is shown in (b).

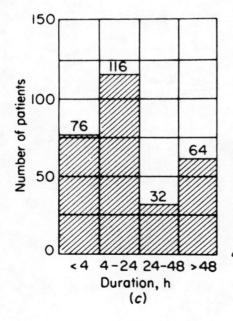

The duration of each headache in hours is shown in (c). From Selby and Lance (100).

Frequency and Duration

Naturally, any study of migraine drawing on data from a neurological clinic includes patients with more severe migraine than those commonly encountered in general practice. More than half the patients attending a clinic were subject to between one and four attacks each month (see Figure 5.2b). The 15 percent of patients who were having more than ten attacks each month were usually anxious or depressed, and it became difficult for both patient and doctor to differentiate between the milder migraine attacks and the more severe forms of tension headache. This is the gray area that makes the classification of headache so difficult. Some severely afflicted patients may awaken each day with migraine headache. Others run a cyclical pattern, having attacks several times a week for about six weeks, each cycle recurring up to five times each year. Most migraine headaches last for twenty-four hours or less (see Figure 5.2c).

6

WHAT CAUSES MIGRAINE?

Where Does the Headache Come From?

The throbbing nature of the headache when migraine is severe suggests that arteries in the head are extremely sensitive to pain when the vessels distend as blood pulses through them. With each heartbeat the pain becomes momentarily worse. It has been known for a long time that pressure over the carotid artery, one of the large arteries one can feel pulsating in the neck (see Figure 6.1), eases the pain of migraine headache once the flow of blood to the head is reduced. In 1796, Erasmus Darwin, the grandfather of the great Charles Darwin, suggested a study using centrifugal force, which, as he quaintly intimated, "cannot be done in private practice, and which I therefore recommend to some hospital physician" (114). He speculated, "What might be the consequence of whirling a person with his head next to centre of motion, so as to force the blood from the brain into the other parts of the body? Would a circulating bed remove any kind of headache?" This challenge was taken up by Dr. Harold G. Wolff 150 years later, using a man-carrying centrifuge (114). He found that rotating a patient with the head centrally placed and the feet positioned outward completely eliminated migraine headache in four patients when they were exposed to a force equivalent to twice that of gravity. Headaches caused by hunger and concussion were also relieved by centrifuging, showing that they too resulted from dilatation of blood vessels.

Wolff continued his observations by studying the effects of stimulating exposed scalp arteries of volunteers who remained

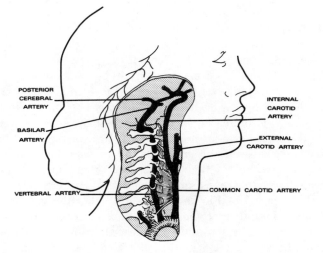

6.1 *Arteries of the head and neck. The main artery that one feels pulsating in the front of the neck is the common carotid artery. This branches into the internal carotid artery, which supplies the brain with blood, and the external carotid artery (crosshatched), which supplies blood to the face and scalp. The vertebral arteries run up to the hindbrain through canals in the cervical vertebrae, where they unite to form the basilar artery.*

conscious and described their sensations. When an artery was distended by stretching its wall with a clamp placed inside the vessel, the subject felt pain in the area over the artery. Threads were then attached to the wall of the artery and pulled rhythmically, so that a throb of pain was felt every time the artery was widened. This procedure was then carried out at two points on the temporal artery; the throbbing pain extended from in front of the ear to the forehead, and the subject started to feel nauseated. This experiment closely simulated the pain of migraine, and the stoic subjects are to be congratulated if not envied for their contribution to scientific knowledge.

If dilatation of the blood vessels causes headache, why do we not get one every time we take a hot bath or play a game of tennis? Most people don't. After exercise or other forms of body heating, the arteries are certainly distended. We can feel their increased pulsation by placing our fingers in front of each ear. The face is flushed and veins on the forehead stand out, showing that blood is flowing freely through the skin and vessels underlying it into the draining veins. Blood does not bank up in the arteries. However, in migraine the face is usually pale. Blood flow is bypassing the skin, but it is not known whether the pressure is increased in the dilated scalp arteries. We do know that these arteries are more sensitive to pain than usual, probably because of the accumulation of chemical substances around them. Wolff found a substance resembling bradykinin around the scalp arteries during migraine headache. Professor Federigo Sicuteri of Florence has shown that the combination of bradykinin and serotonin will produce pain in blood vessels, and we know that serotonin is released from its body stores during migraine attacks (101). We thus have a simple hypothesis: The arteries of migraine are painful when dilated because they are sensitized by bradykinin and serotonin.

New Thoughts on Headache

The hypothesis set out above cannot be the complete answer. Dr. Peter Drummond and I examined a series of patients while they had a migraine headache and found that the headache could be eased in one-third of the cases by pressing the temporal artery, the pulse in front of the ear, on the same side as the headache (31). In those patients whose pain was relieved by applying pressure, recordings from the scalp arteries showed an increase in pulsation during headache. Thermograms, pictures taken with a heat-sensitive camera, demonstrated areas of increased heat loss over dilated arteries in the affected temple (see Figure 6.2). In another one-third of patients, the headache was eased by pressure over the carotid artery on the same side of the neck, but in the remaining one-third the headache continued unabated in spite of the interrupted blood flow to that part of the head. The vessels may continue to send pain impulses even when they are not distended, or perhaps there is a central factor as well, such as an opening of the pain gate as described in chapter 2.

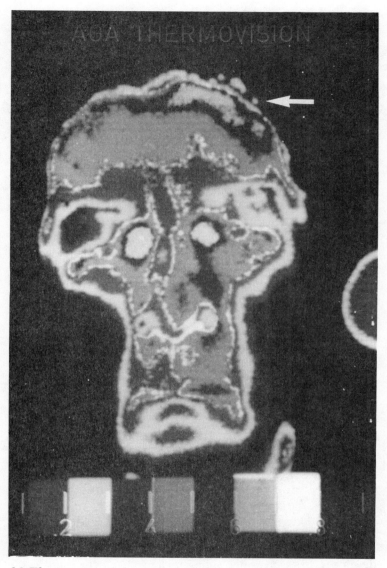

6.2 *Thermogram of the face taken during a migraine headache. The area in the left upper forehead and temple, designated by the arrow, is a "hot spot," indicating dilatation of blood vessels in this region. The outline of the face can be made out with the exception of the outer cheeks, which are too cool to register. Squares at the bottom indicate skin temperature (color-coded in the original photograph).*

Nerve impulses pass from the large arteries of the brain along the trigeminal nerve (Figure 2.2). Dr. M. A. Moskowitz and his colleagues at Massachusetts General Hospital, Boston, have found that the trigeminal nerve contains serotonin and substance P, a peptide that is thought to be a neurotransmitter for the perception of pain and that is also a potent dilator of blood vessels (85). He postulates that substance P might leak from the nerve terminals around the blood vessels of the brain, causing them to dilate and ache. In our own laboratory, Dr. Geoff Lambert has found that activity in the trigeminal nerve sets up a reflex that increases flow in the arteries of the face and scalp, suggesting that the pain of migraine could cause blood vessels to dilate instead of the dilated vessels producing pain (61). Dr. Peter Goadsby and Dr. Graham Macdonald of the Prince Henry Hospital, Sydney, showed that this dilator reflex depends on the release of another peptide, vasoactive intestinal polypeptide (VIP)—so called because it was first found in the intestines (43). The plot has now thickened with the discovery that these peptides affect the blood vessels to the brain and scalp. It is possible that the primary event in common migraine is a spontaneous discharge of the trigeminal nerve pathways inside the brain and that the release of substance P from trigeminal nerve branches adds a vascular component to the pain. Reflex connections from the trigeminal nerve could cause similar changes in the face and scalp by the release of VIP.

The Significance of Ice-Cream Headache and Ice-Pick Pains in Migraine

Even in periods of freedom from migraine, migrainous subjects carry with them a susceptibility to head pain. Drummond and I found that one-third of the migrainous patients who developed headache after eating ice cream felt the pain in the same part of the head that was affected by their migraine attacks (33). Moreover, 42 percent of migrainous patients are prone to sudden jabs of pain in the head ("ice-pick pains"), compared with only 3 percent of nonheadache subjects. We found that ice-pick pains coincided with the site of the customary migraine headache in 40 percent of cases. It therefore appears that the trigeminal pathways may discharge momentarily to cause ice-pick pains or may become active for seconds or minutes after cooling of the pharynx to cause ice-cream headaches. It is possible that the same pathways could fire off spontaneously for hours or days to cause the pain of migraine headaches.

How Do You Explain the Flashing Lights?

Classical migraine is distinguished by a prodrome or aura lasting up to sixty minutes, in which the unfortunate subjects see flashing lights or zigzag "fortification spectra." They may also feel odd prickling sensations around the mouth or in the limbs. They may feel weak, or their speech may become incoherent. It has long been suspected that blood flow to the brain was impaired during the prodrome, a suspicion that has been confirmed by modern medical techniques, although it is still not certain whether active constriction of blood vessels causes the cerebral symptoms or whether the nerve cells in the cerebral cortex cease to function and the blood flow diminishes as a result.

In 1936, Dr. A. M. Goltman described the strange fluctuations in size of the brain during migraine attacks in a woman who had a bone defect in her skull (44). The pressure inside the skull could be judged by whether the scalp was bulging over the bone defect or was sunken inward. Goltman noted, "Immediately before the onset of the headache attack her face appeared blanched, at which time there was a definite depression at the site of the bone defect." Then as the headache developed, "the skull depression began to fill up, and ultimately the intracranial contents protruded, assuming the appearance of a tumour. When it thus became a bulging mass it was not tender and did not pulsate on palpation. The patient then began to vomit. The pallor of the face gave way to a flush. After twelve to seventy-three hours the headache subsided and the intracranial contents resumed their former relation to the bone defect."

More specific information has come from X rays of the blood vessels taken during migraine and from studies of blood flow using radioactive isotopes. It is possible to obtain clear pictures of the arteries supplying the brain by injecting them with a material that does not transmit X rays, so that the whole arterial tree can be seen in silhouette. Such X rays (called arteriograms or angiograms) taken during the early phase of migraine, while visual and other sensory disturbances are in progress, have shown that the large arteries are usually normal in appearance. This suggests that it is only the smaller branches, not seen in the arteriogram, that constrict in this phase.

The electroencephalogram (EEG), which records the electrical "brain waves," shows an abnormal pattern in the area of the brain where the symptoms arise. When radioactive Xenon gas is inhaled or injected into the arteries, the passage of blood through different parts of the brain may be measured accurately by detectors placed on the head. These techniques have shown that blood flow is reduced by up to 50 percent in the parts of the brain that are giving rise to symptoms. When cerebral symptoms disappear and headache follows, the blood flow *increases* by about 20 percent in classical migraine. This increased blood flow is not responsible for headache. Jes Olesen and his colleagues in Copenhagen have shown that in patients with classical migraine the headache may start while blood flow is still diminished, and that the flow may not alter in patients with common migraine (86, 87). Pictures taken of the brain by a special X-ray technique known as computerized axial tomography (CT or CAT scanning) demonstrate swelling of the brain in some cases of classical migraine.

Brain function slows down before and during migraine headache. Studies using a new radioisotope technique, positron emission tomography (PET scanning), have shown that the brain uses 10 to 30 percent less oxygen at these times (98). This may lead to a secondary reduction in cerebral blood flow, since blood flow alters automatically to supply the brain with the precise amount of oxygen it needs.

One facet that has not been previously explained is the slow spread of sensory disturbances in some patients. Zigzags of light may appear in one part of the visual field and slowly move across the field, leaving patchy or complete loss of vision behind them. Dr. K. S. Lashley, a distinguished Harvard psychologist who was subject to this sort of visual hallucination, retained his spirit of scientific inquiry despite the advancing migrainous eclipse (70). He sat in front of a dark screen on many occasions, meticulously plotting the extent of his field of vision by sticking pins into the screen to mark its outer limits. As the perimeters of his vision shrank he constructed a series of contour lines on the screen to help him later determine the rate at which his sight had decreased. He calculated that the cortex of his brain must have been thrown out of action by some process that moved across its surface at the speed of three millimeters each minute.

Now it so happens that there is a process well known to physiologists that executes a slow march across the cortex at precisely three millimeters per minute, called spreading depression, caused by a change in the membrane of nerve cells. Moreover, it is preceded by a constriction of small vessels and is followed by their dilatation. It seems highly probable that this process underlies the gradual onset of the cerebral symptoms many patients experience, the slow growth of numbness over one side of the body, the plucking out one by one of the words required for coherent speech, and the progressive suffocation of the intellect that is a transient but disturbing part of the migraine syndrome in some patients.

Meticulous observations by Olesen and his colleagues in Copenhagen demonstrated that blood flow is diminished during the prodrome of classical migraine, starting at the back of the brain in the visual cortex and spreading slowly over the cerebral cortex at the rate of two to three millimeters per minute. This accords well with the clinical findings of Lashley and the data on spreading depression (see Figure 6.3).

Why should the visual symptoms sometimes comprise flashes or pinpoints of light and sometimes shimmering or jittering zigzags of color? Experimental work has provided some insight into this problem.

Dr. D. H. Hubel and Dr. T. N. Wiesel of the department of

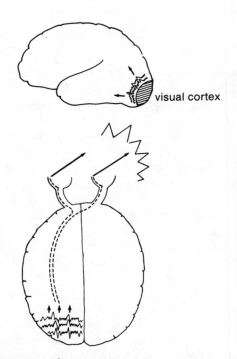

visual cortex

6.3 *Mechanism of fortification spectra. A wave of excitation spreads forward over the visual cortex. Because the visual pathways from eye to brain are crossed (dotted lines), a disturbance of the left side of the brain causes flashing lights or zigzags to be seen in the right field of vision.*

neurobiology, Harvard University, have shown that the visual cortex is arranged in sheets or columns of cells, each of which responds selectively to a bar of light held at a certain angle in front of the eye (53). As the angle of the bar is slowly rotated, one column of cells after another is thrown into activity. If we imagine the reverse of this process, any stimulation of a column of brain cells would cause a person to "see" a bar of light at a certain angle to the horizontal. If a wave of excitation crept over the visual cortex, the patient would see a succession of bars of light at different angles shimmering or jittering as column after column was stimulated. This is what happens in migraine. A wave of excitation sweeps over the cortex causing symptoms like zigzag lights in front of the eyes, followed by a period of depression of vision when the patient cannot see clearly.

If, on the other hand, the whole visual cortex is irritated at once by a generalized reduction in blood flow, the cells at the outer end of each column (farthest away from the source of blood supply) would fire off singly or in groups, giving the impression of stars or flashes of light rather than bars or zigzags. This is a common experience with some migraine patients. Dr. G. S. Brindley and Dr. B. S. Lewin of University College, London, stimulated the visual cortex of blind people by electrodes in an attempt to reproduce a pattern of vision that the patient can "see." The patients reported seeing fine points of white light like distant stars in the sky (20). We therefore have a plausible explanation for the visual symptoms of migraine, depending on whether the cortical function is impaired diffusely and simultaneously or progressively by a process spreading sideways over the surface.

What could be responsible for constriction of small vessels and the associated changes in cortical function? It could be peculiar to the blood vessels themselves, say in response to head injury, or as a reaction to some chemical substance in the bloodstream, or the direct result of a discharge along nerve pathways from the brain stem.

Around A.D. 100 Aretaeus, a physician practicing in Alexandria, pointed out that patients with migraine "flee the light; the darkness soothes their disease" (2). Why should patients with migraine wish to flee from the light and seek refuge in a darkened room? It was thought that aversion to light (photophobia) was caused by changes in the blood vessels in the white of the eye, as these vessels commonly constrict in the early stages of an attack and dilate later on so that the eye appears bloodshot. Another theory involved irritation of the nerve supply to the eye from the pain of migraine. Neither of these explanations is completely satisfactory, for many patients also become acutely aware of smells and sounds. Smells that might be pleasing under normal circumstances may be perceived as an unbearable stench at the height of migraine headache, and background noise that customarily passes unnoticed may seem intolerable. There is surely a lowering of activity in the nervous connections that normally modify perception from the special senses so that incoming information becomes magnified in migraine. Professor Federigo Sicuteri postulated that this is caused by the loss of a chemical substance, serotonin, which is employed in transmission of nerve impulses between some nerve cells (102). He believes that the absence of serotonin also reduces the influence of the pain-control pathway (discussed in chapter 2) and thus makes the person more aware of pain, so that ordinary background sensations give rise to a feeling of pain during migraine headache.

Nausea and vomiting are distressing symptoms of migraine at some time for most patients. Abdominal pain and diarrhea may also occur. It is quite common for people to remark on disturbances of appetite or bowel function immediately before the attack. It seems that the whole gastrointestinal tract is stilled before migraine starts—the calm before the storm. As the attack gathers momentum, waves of contraction are stirred up in the gastrointestinal tract, reaching their climax in vomiting and sometimes diarrhea as well. Any explanation for this behavior cannot be based on the pain of migraine, because nausea may precede the headache. It could be caused by the vomiting center in the brain stem or by the release of serotonin, that jack-of-all-trades, ubiquitous and potent, into the bloodstream. It is known that 95 percent of serotonin in the body is contained in the wall of the intestine and that the administration of serotonin increases intestinal activity. We also know that diarrhea is a major symptom of a carcinoid tumor, and carcinoid tumors manufacture large amounts of serotonin. It is possible that serotonin, which we know is released from its body stores during migraine, may be responsible for vomiting and diarrhea. This overactivity of the gastrointestinal tract may in turn release more serotonin from its hiding place in the intestinal wall.

What about the fluid retention that often accompanies migraine headache? Finger rings become tight, ankles swell noticeably, the face appears puffy—all these are signs of fluid retention. As the migraine attack wears off, large volumes of pale urine may be passed, thus eliminating excessive water from the body. At the risk of oversimplification, serotonin is also a possible cause of fluid retention, because it can alter filtration in the kidney so that fluid is conserved in the body. Other hormones from the pituitary or adrenal glands can have the same effect.

Nerves or Chemicals?

Emotion can induce migraine within minutes. A patient of mine was having a heated argument with a girl friend about the rebellious attitude he had toward his father when he had been a teenager, a subject that had distressed him in later years. At the height of the argument his vision started to blur, and soon he could see only the center of objects. This tunnel vision lasted for about ten minutes, after which his characteristic migraine headache developed. Some weeks later he was attending a cinema and found that the film dealt with the same problem of the father–son relationship that had always troubled him. The same sensation of distress swept over him. Within a few minutes his vision misted over, and tunnel vision was again followed by a headache.

What is the link between mind and body? Is the sequence of constriction and dilatation of blood vessels brought about by nerve pathways or by chemical messengers in the bloodstream? In A.D. 600, Paul of Aegina, a Greek physician at the medical school of Alexandria, wrote, "Headache, which is one of the most serious complaints, is sometimes occasioned by an intemperament solely, sometimes by a redundance of humors, and sometimes by both" (1).

Until ten years ago it seemed unlikely that the brain could control cerebral blood vessels directly, because the known connections (sympathetic and parasympathetic nerves) could be cut without preventing further migraine headaches. It was known that the blood levels of monoamines, such as serotonin and norepinephrine, increased before migraine attacks and dropped during the headache phase (5). It was thought that these substances could constrict small vessels and then, as their blood level dropped, permit a passive dilatation of larger vessels.

Serotonin is carried in blood platelets, which clump together early in migraine and release their serotonin. Clumps of platelets further interfere with blood flow through the cerebral circulation and can lead to clotting in the arteries, prolonging symptoms beyond the migraine attack and perhaps causing a stroke (complicated migraine). The released serotonin could act with other substances surrounding the vessels, like bradykinin, causing them to ache.

If this were the case, one would have to postulate that the release of serotonin takes place habitually in one part of the circulation, because the symptoms are often consistent in a particular patient—for example, left-sided blurring of vision and left-sided numbness. This would seem unlikely enough. Even if this did happen, why would the ensuing headache often involve the inappropriate side of the head? In the example given above, left-sided symptoms must originate in the right side of the brain because the connections are crossed, yet the headache in such a person is as often left-sided as right-sided. Serotonin may still play a part in sensitizing vessels and in inducing other symptoms of migraine, but it now seems unlikely that it could be the primary mediator unless blood levels are reflecting changes in the brain where serotonin acts as a neurotransmitter in the pain-control pathway (see chapter 2).

Could migraine be a direct reaction of the blood vessels themselves? Migraine may be brought on by heat and exercise, alcohol, or drugs that dilate blood vessels, as well as by the injection of substances into the arteries for X-ray examinations (arteriography). Even in these instances, there is a lag of anywhere from minutes to hours before headache develops, so there is plenty of time for the nervous system to come into the picture.

In some cases, there seems little doubt that the nervous system is directly involved. Looking at light reflected from rippling water may bring on a migraine initiated by a disturbance of vision. The vigorous use of one arm can lead to numbness and tingling of that arm as a prodrome to migraine. It is probable that the nervous system is overreactive in migrainous subjects and responds rapidly to any intense bombardment of the brain by sensory impulses or emotional disturbance.

Why Is Migraine Headache Usually One-Sided?

Over the past ten years new pathways have been discovered that enable the brain to control its own blood supply. Areas in the brain stem rich in serotonin (raphe nuclei) and norepinephrine (locus ceruleus) have been shown to send bundles of nerve fibers upward through the brain which then branch out and are distributed to all areas of the cerebral cortex (see Figure 6.4). The locus ceruleus, or "blue spot," is particularly interesting, because it can damp down the activity of brain cells and reduce the blood flow to them. Work in our own laboratory by Peter Goadsby and others has shown that these changes affect mainly the half of the brain on the side stimulated (42). If the locus is stimulated more rapidly, it can then increase blood flow in the vessels of the face and head by a reflex in the same way that excitation of the trigeminal nerve increases blood flow (61). So here we have a possible mechanism for shutting down the activity of the cortex on one side of the brain, reducing its blood flow, and later increasing the flow to structures outside the brain in the face and scalp, changes closely resembling those of classical migraine. Remember that the same brain-stem structures are involved in the pain-control system (Figures 2.2, 2.3), so that they may play a key role in both the neurological symptoms and the headache of migraine (Figure 6.4).

Conclusions

Migraine is a hereditary disorder in which certain bodily systems employing monoamines, such as serotonin and norepinephrine, appear to be in a hypersensitive state, reacting promptly and excessively to stimuli such as emotion, bombardment with sensory impulses, or any sudden change in the internal or external environment. If the brain-stem systems controlling the cerebral cortex become active, the brain starts to shut down, a process starting at the back of the brain in the visual cortex and working slowly forward. The pain nucleus of the trigeminal nerve becomes spontaneously active; pain is felt in the head or upper neck and blood flow in the face and

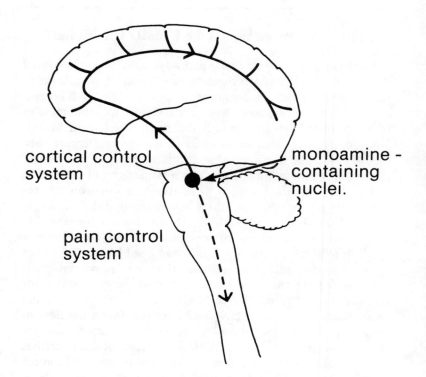

cortical control
system

monoamine -
containing
nuclei.

pain control
system

6.4 *Upward and downward projections from the brain stem. Areas of the brain stem, such as the locus ceruleus, send fibers up to the cerebral cortex, regulating the activity of brain cells and their blood supply. Descending fibers are part of the pain-control system. Either or both of these systems may play a part in migraine.*

scalp increases reflexively. Norepinephrine is released from the adrenal gland and causes the platelets that release serotonin to clump. Serotonin in the circulation interacts with bradykinin and peptides such as substance P present in the tissues around the vessels to increase their sensibility to pain.

The brain-stem nuclei of one side have a reciprocal effect on those of the other side; their effects may alternate, causing cortical changes on one side and headache on the other, or causing the headache itself to change from side to side.

This is the present hypothesis for the mechanism by which migrainous symptoms are produced (69). Although we have examined in detail how the brain works, we must not lose sight of the fact that migraine involves the person as an individual: brain, mind, and life-style. Treatment must be aimed at both mind and body. In spite of this, the detailed dissection we have undertaken is not solely of academic interest. Many of the treatments for migraine are aimed at altering the function of the monoamine systems we have considered, and they do so with considerable success.

7

THE TREATMENT
OF MIGRAINE

There are many who never seek attention for their headaches because they believe that nothing can be done to help them. There are others who believe that if they take a pill whenever a headache becomes too severe, they have done all that is humanly possible, whether it works or not, and that they must then put up with their headache for hours or even days at a time. Much is known about migraine and much can be done about it. Migraine does not destroy life, but it can destroy the joy of living. Treatment starts with the consideration of the patient as well as the disease.

A Patient Is a Person

We have seen that the migraine patient is not subject to more stresses than other people but reacts more intensely to them. While there may be some advantage in reducing the stresses from without, the logical approach is to try to strengthen the resistance to stress from within. It is first necessary for patients to know themselves and to stand back and view themselves objectively.

What are your internal resources, your strengths, and are you using them to the best advantage? Are you using your abilities to help others in the family and in the community, or are you swamping them in self-pity because you are concentrating only on your inadequacies, your illness, and your disappointments? Do you have a clear goal in life, one worth achieving? If so, do you have the ability to achieve it? Is it a realistic goal? Will it give you happiness or bring happiness to others? What is the most logical approach to success, and how can you best work toward it? Some time occasionally spent in this form of constructive introspection may save much time and trouble in the long run. There is the well-known story of the airplane captain who announced that he had bad news. "The navigator has lost his way and we do not know where we are going. However, I also have good news. We have a tail wind and are making excellent progress."

We must live and work in the present, and, to the best of our ability, be content with our day-to-day lives. But the present must also be used for planning an acceptable future. I believe that everyone needs some sort of goal and that to live for the day is not enough for most people. In what way can you positively change your daily routine? Would a different job, a different environment for living or working, a different approach to life give you the stimulus you seek?

There are times, of course, when so many problems arise that it is possible only to tackle each day as it comes. Then, when things ease up a little, the times comes again for further stock-taking, renewed motivation, and an upsurge of activity. Along with the broad view of the future, there must be some resting places along the way, some small pleasures to enhance each day or each week. I would urge you to take time off for a hobby, an afternoon away from the children, or a quiet drink at the end of the day. Exercising, going to the movies, or planning a vacation can help prevent the internal pressure from rising to dangerous levels. This is particularly important for women who have chosen to stay home with their small children but feel permanently housebound, without any breaks in their routine and with few of the daily contacts that provide stimulation for those who work in the world outside the home.

Finally, the process of introspection must include one's personal inadequacies. In what way do you not measure up to your own expectations and those of your husband or wife, children, and friends? If there is some serious personal problem involving social, sexual, or business relationships, or just coping with general daily chores, you would benefit from discussing these with your family doctor, who may refer you to a psychiatrist. Discussing a problem, particularly with someone trained in counseling, may reveal a solution that has not occurred to you. If there are a series of minor problems that are a recurring cause of anxiety, analyzing them will help you learn to cope with them one at a time. If the problem is beyond your own resources, you may be helped by formal psychotherapy.

The results of an interesting combined approach were reported by Sydney psychologists K. R. Mitchell and D. M. Mitchell, from the University of New South Wales, in the treatment of patients with migraine (81). They started with the premise that the reduction of migraine frequency depended on the ability to control emotional reactions, and they prepared two programs to compare their effectiveness. In the first program, relaxation training was followed by the application of this training to the tension-producing situations peculiar to the individual. The second treatment group went on to desensitization procedures, which included making a graded list of anxiety-producing stimuli, evoking these by imagery, and pairing each stimulus with a relaxed state. A further stage was "assertiveness therapy," in which the subjects underwent training in acting out their feelings of love, affection, or hostility in socially acceptable and appropriate forms. Various difficulties, such as sexual problems, were explained and discussed. While the level of anxiety did not drop appreciably during the thirty-two-week treatment period, the second group, with combined relaxation, desensitization, and assertiveness therapy, showed significant reduction in the frequency and severity of migraine attacks in contrast to the other group.

Patients may be helped by any means of relaxation for mind and body. Some may benefit from yoga or Transcendental Meditation. There is little doubt that the ideal treatment for migraine includes both psychological and physical measures.

The Way of Life

The common factor in the wide variety of precipitants of migraine appears to be the *rate of change* within the body or its environment. This can be as direct as a blow on the head or as indirect as sleeping late on Sunday morning. If the only aim in life were to prevent migraine, either a life of unrelieved monotony or one maintained at a steady pitch of feverish excitement would be the solution. Since neither is practical or desirable, some compromise has to be worked out, avoiding as much as possible sudden peaks and valleys in emotional pitch. This is largely a matter of common sense *and planning.* The working day should be organized to run as smoothly as possible, with the work load spread evenly over each day and over each week. On the weekend, there is no need to let everything slump. A radical change of pace from constant tension to complete relaxation is a sure way to ensure that the weekend is spoiled by a headache. Sleeping in is a particularly pernicious habit for many and is to be avoided by all prone to "weekend migraine."

Anything found to be a trigger factor should obviously be eliminated whenever possible. Missing meals, drinking red wines, or eating certain foods affect only certain people, and each individual must find out which, if any, of these factors applies to him or her. A few people get their headaches only after rigorous exercise, but this does not mean that all exercise is forbidden. On the contrary, regular exercise accustoms the blood vessels to a normal sequence of dilatation rather than the incongruous combination of dilatation and constriction that takes place in migraine. It has been said that standing on the head induces a reflex vasoconstriction of scalp arteries that is beneficial in migraine and that may actually abort an attack if the patient is astute enough to detect the early symptoms, agile enough to do a headstand, and devoid of the embarrassment this custom may cause!

Diet

The possibility of dietary factors precipitating migraine headache was discussed in chapter 5. There is a strong tradition of folklore and anecdotal experience testifying to the importance of certain foods in the genesis of migraine, but hard data are lacking. Dr. Jose Medina and Dr. Seymour Diamond of the

Chicago Medical School compared the headache frequency of migrainous patients on a diet rich in amines (such as aged cheeses and chocolate) and permitting alcohol intake with a diet avoiding these substances, each study lasting for six weeks (79). The headache frequency was no different from that recorded on the normal diet.

In 1980, Dr. Jean Monro and her colleagues from the National Hospital for Nervous Diseases and the Middlesex Hospital in London studied forty-seven migrainous patients over a period of two years, during which time fourteen patients dropped out (84). Of the remaining thirty-three, food culprits were identified in twenty-three, and elimination of these foods from the diet was said to result in relief (complete in most cases), usually within two weeks. No details were given of headache frequencies or length of follow-up. A correlation was found between the suspected foods and the presence in the patients' blood of antibodies that reacted to those specific foods (radioallergosorbent or RAST test).

Even more startling results were claimed by Dr. J. Egger and a group from the Great Ormond St. Childrens Hospital, London, who reported that 93 percent of eighty-eight children with severe, frequent migraine recovered on diets from which provocative foods had been removed (35). Not only were their headaches relieved, but behavior disorder, abdominal pain, asthma, eczema, and epileptic fits were also said to improve. These results may not be generally applicable, because the group of children studied was unusual. Over half the children suffered from allergic diseases, almost half had behavior disturbances, and even between attacks of migraine fourteen out of the eighty-eight were subject to epilepsy, and six had signs of damage to the nervous system. Further studies on more typical groups of migrainous adults and children are clearly required.

In the meantime, it is obviously sensible for anyone to avoid foods that appear to trigger his attacks, whether the sensitivity is physical or psychological, inherent or conditioned. There is certainly no need, based on our present knowledge, for a blanket ban of chocolate, fatty foods, oranges, or any other component of one's diet.

Physical Measures

What physical treatment may be helpful? The age-old method of massaging the scalp or neck muscles, which contract reflexly in migraine, often gives considerable relief. Relaxation exercises (outlined in chapter 8) will also help in reducing the frequency of migraine attacks. Any method that aids in relaxation, whether it be formal exercise, biofeedback, meditation, yoga, or hypnosis, may decrease the frequency of migraine.

The application of hot or cold packs is another time-honored remedy that merits closer study. In theory, cold packs placed over the large arteries, such as those in the temples, should constrict them and reduce the intensity of the headache. Hot packs are used to dilate the small peripheral vessels to flush the skin and permit the free flow of blood through them. Some say that a long, hot shower followed by a cold shower may abort a headache.

Biofeedback

The term "biofeedback" is used for a variety of techniques that give the subject information about bodily reactions, which may then be altered by an effort of will. For example, wires can be attached to the skin over muscles of the forehead or temples so that the electrical activity generated by contracting muscles can be amplified and displayed on a meter or video screen. Alternatively, muscle activity can be transformed into a sound that gets louder as the muscles contract (see Figure 7.1). In either case, subjects have a guide to help them determine the degree of muscle contraction that helps in their relaxation program. Other devices measure forehead and hand temperature while subjects think of their hands getting warmer. The pulsation of arteries in the temples can be recorded so that subjects can try to diminish the amplitude of pulsation. Some researchers consider one method superior to another in reducing the tendency to headache, but the consensus of opinion seems to be that all methods help promote relaxation, although they may be no more beneficial for migraine than relaxation therapy alone.

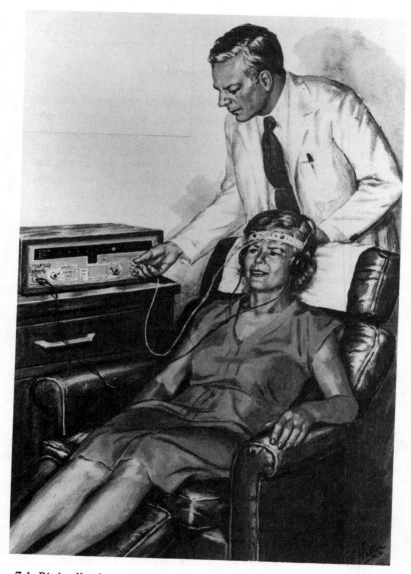

7.1 *Biofeedback. One method of biofeedback records the contraction of scalp muscles and transforms the intensity of the contraction to a sound played back to the patient through earphones. The sound's intensity decreases as the patient relaxes. Illustration courtesy of Dr. Frank Netter and the* CIBA *Pharmaceutical Company, reproduced from* Clinical Symposia, *Vol. 33, number 2, 1981.*

Acupuncture

Many of the traditional Chinese acupuncture points are in areas of the head and neck that become tender during migraine headache. Injection of a local anesthetic agent into these areas, or even dry needling of the tender spots in muscle, can relieve headache temporarily, probably because of the interaction of pain impulses from the head and neck described in chapter 2.

In 1984, Dr. L. Loh and a team of neurologists from the National Hospital for Nervous Diseases, London, reported the result of a study of acupuncture therapy in forty-one patients suffering from migraine or tension headache who had not responded previously to medication (74). After three months, sixteen patients showed moderate or great improvement, eight reported slight improvement, and seventeen were unchanged. Of twenty-nine patients who switched from acupuncture to medical treatment, most preferred acupuncture, which was not surprising since they had already failed to respond to medical treatment. Some 45 percent of patients derived no benefit from either form of therapy.

Acupuncture is time-consuming for both patient and doctor and can be quite unpleasant for the patient. It is safe, providing that adequately sterilized or disposable needles are used; otherwise there is an unacceptable risk of transmission of a form of liver disease (hepatitis B) and acquired immune deficiency syndrome (AIDS) from patient to patient. It should be considered for patients who do not improve with conventional treatment.

Manipulation of the Neck

The question of the treatment of migraine never comes up for discussion without someone claiming that manipulation of the neck is an infallible cure. Certainly any cervical disturbances should be adequately treated, just as it is important to eliminate any other known trigger factor in migraine. My own experience is that manipulation of the neck benefits only a limited number of patients. Many patients whom I see have already had their necks manipulated by doctors or chiropractors without any significant change in their headache pattern. The late Dr. James Cyriax of St. Thomas's Hospital, London, stated that an "attack of migraine can sometimes be instantly aborted by strong traction on the neck. Half a minute's traction in some cases is regularly successful, in others not." He goes on to say, "A minority of patients have reported to me, some years after the reduction by manipulation, that since that time attacks of obvious migraine have ceased." He noted such improvement only in middle-aged patients—not in the young (26). I remain skeptical about any specific role for neck disturbance in migraine and the advantages to be obtained from manipulation of the neck.

An evaluation of manipulation of the neck for the relief of migraine was undertaken by Gordon Parker and others from the University of New South Wales, Sydney (88). Migraine sufferers were divided randomly into three groups. One group was treated by chiropractic manipulation, a second group was manipulated by doctors or physiotherapists, and a third group had a course of "mobilization" of the neck (gentle movements within the normal range of the neck joints). Migraine symptoms were reduced by 28 percent in all groups over a six-month period, but the severity of headaches was less in the group treated by chiropractic methods. It is interesting to note that a follow-up twenty months after the course of treatment showed that migraine attacks had diminished by a further 19 percent. This probably represents the natural history of the disorder, since patients usually seek treatment when symptoms are at their worst and improvement is thus likely whatever form of therapy is employed.

Surgical Treatment

Operations on sympathetic and parasympathetic nerve pathways have not proven to be of benefit in migraine. Coagulating or dividing the trigeminal nerve provides some relief from pain but has the disadvantages of making one side of the face numb and causing the patient to lose the protective blink reflex on the same side, so that the eye can easily become infected. For this reason the operation is considered only as a last resort, and then only for those patients whose headaches habitually affect the same side of the head.

Sometimes localized procedures can be helpful. In those people whose pain is limited to one side of the forehead and is relieved by an injection of local anesthetic around the forehead nerves, cutting those nerves can provide short-term or lasting benefit. Similarly, if the pain always starts in one side of the back of the head or is limited to that area, injection of the region with local anesthetic and a long-acting form of cortisone may temporarily relieve discomfort, and sectioning the appropriate nerve may then give an even longer period of relief. If the headaches started after an injury to the scalp and are restricted to the injured area, surgical removal of the nerves and vessels from that region of the scalp can foster permanent improvement. At present, however, surgery does not offer much hope to most sufferers from migraine.

Histamine Sensitization

An old method of treating migraine is to give increasing doses of histamine, a potent dilator of cranial arteries, in the hope of desensitizing them to other dilator influences. Unfortunately, histamine acts on the intracranial arteries more than on the scalp arteries, which are partly responsible for the migraine headache. There is no evidence that a general release of histamine causes migraine, but the histamine level does increase slightly in the blood after the attack, suggesting that it may be released locally at the site of the headache. The antihistamine drugs in present use do little to prevent migraine. A new group of antihistamines that block histamine-2 receptors (a different histamine action on blood vessels) is equally ineffective.

The technique of histamine desensitization involves daily injections of histamine, increasing progressively in dosage, or three intravenous infusions at weekly intervals. (An infusion is a slow injection of a solution into a vein by a drip apparatus given over a period of hours.) The latter method has the advantage that the patient's reaction can be observed closely. The object of this method is to run the intravenous drip at a speed sufficient to induce flushing of the face but not enough to provoke headache. When Dr. George Selby and I analyzed results of this treatment in the 1960s, we found after eight months that 21 percent of the patients had remained free of headache and 42 percent were substantially improved (100). It is questionable whether the results warrant the time and inconvenience involved, but it can be used for patients not responding to other treatments.

Hormonal Therapy and Fluid Retention

Because of the fluid and salt retention that accompanies migraine, and that can also be a prominent feature in the days preceding menstruation, salt restriction has been advocated, along with diuretics that help eliminate salt from the body. Fluid and salt retention can certainly be prevented, and this may relieve unpleasant symptoms such as distension of the abdomen and swelling of the face, fingers, and ankles. Regrettably, it does not usually prevent migraine.

The discovery that the fall in estrogen levels initiates premenstrual migraine has renewed interest in the possibilities of hormonal treatment. Different dosages, combinations, and sequences of synthetic estrogens and progesterones have been used in the various forms of the contraceptive pill, and these have been studied to see if they will prevent premenstrual migraine. While some pills reduce the incidence of headache, and an occasional patient may lose her headaches on a particular pill, the majority find that menstrual migraine continues to appear predictably. Treatment with synthetic progestogenic agents has proved disappointing. Implanting estrogen tablets under the skin has been advocated, but further study is needed to see if this method is generally applicable.

Stopping the Acute Attack

If migraine recurs only infrequently or if it appears at predictable times, such as the day before menstruation starts or

Sunday morning when one is lying in bed, then it is simple enough to take the appropriate medication at the first sign of an attack. When a sufferer awakens regularly with a fully developed headache, its occurrence can often be analyzed and prevented in the future by taking a pill the night before. This can be done if the patient predictably feels elated the day before an attack or has some other identifiable warning. For children, one or two aspirin usually stop the attack from progressing, but there are few adults whose attacks will be halted by any of the commonly used analgesics, including some combinations that have been marketed under brand names which suggest that they are specifically for migraine. An age-old device for easing the pain of migraine is compression of the dilated scalp vessels (see Figure 7.2), but medication will do this more effectively.

Most of the pills prescribed by doctors for treatment of acute attacks of migraine are not painkillers but contain ergotamine tartrate, an agent that constricts the large arteries of the scalp and affects the central nervous system as well, often preventing a migraine attack from developing. For this reason, the dose must be suitable for that individual and the pills taken before the arteries are too dilated. Patients must therefore carry the pills with them so that they can take one or two as soon as the first symptom of an attack appears. If each episode starts with blurring of vision or a similar disturbance, the pills should be taken immediately so that they have sufficient time to constrict the scalp arteries before the situation is irretrievable. If the patient feels nauseated and vomits in the early stages of the attack, there is no point in taking medication orally. Under these circumstances the use of a suppository is logical and effective. Another method that can be used is to inhale a fine powder of ergotamine tartrate deeply into the lungs from a pressure pack or Medihaler.

Some pills consist of ergotamine tartrate alone. Others have caffeine in them because it promotes absorption of ergotamine and increases constriction of the arteries as well as acting as a stimulant. A third group contains an additional agent to diminish nausea.

The following are some of those most commonly employed.

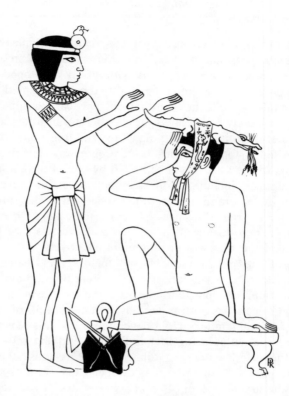

7.2 *The treatment of migraine in 1200* B.C. *A clay crocodile was bound to the head of the patient so that magic herbs could be placed in its mouth. Note that the band compresses the temporal artery. Today, the clay crocodile has been eliminated as a medium, and magic herbs are given directly to the patient. The cartoon was drawn by P. Cunningham and is reproduced by permission of Dr. John Edmeads.*

Ergotamine Tartrate Alone

This is available in uncoated tablets containing one or two milligrams (Wigrettes, Ergomar, Lingraine). Every patient has to determine the suitable dose, sufficient to stop the migraine from developing but not so much as to cause nausea as a side effect. The usual dose is one or two milligrams at the first indication of an attack, repeated in one-half to one hour if necessary. If the headache has not been relieved after the repeated dose, there is no benefit in taking more; indeed it can be dangerous, because excessive amounts can cause whiteness and numbness of the fingers from constriction of the small vessels. The uncoated tablets are said to be well absorbed from the mouth if held under the tongue, but there is some doubt about this, and most of the medication is probably absorbed from the stomach. A traditional way of prescribing ergotamine tablets is to direct that the tablet be taken every hour for up to six hours, but this is not really an effective method because an adequate level of the drug in the bloodstream is not achieved. The most direct way of accomplishing this is by injection, and some patients who do not respond to tablets, suppositories, or a Medihaler can be taught to give themselves an injection. By this route the dosage is lower than if given by mouth, one-quarter to one-half milligram by subcutaneous or intramuscular injection. In many countries, ergotamine is not available for injection; a closely related drug, dihydroergotamine (DHE), is used instead. The usual dose of DHE is one milligram by intramuscular injection.

Compounds Containing Ergotamine Tartrate

Cafergot and Wigraine.   Ergotamine tartrate (one milligram) is combined with caffeine (one hundred milligrams) in Cafergot or Wigraine tablets. One or two tablets are usually given at the onset of the attack and may be repeated. Some people are sensitive to caffeine and may feel unpleasantly overstimulated if more than two tablets are taken. Similar preparations are available as suppositories.

Cafergot P-B and Wigraine-PB suppositories.   These suppositories of ergotamine tartrate contain two milligrams of the active agent as well as caffeine in addition to other agents with a sedative action. The first time these are used it is advisable to cut one in half lengthwise (after cooling it in the refrigerator) and insert only one-half, because some patients notice cramps in the legs after using the full dose contained in the suppository. Once it is established that the suppositories are well tolerated, one may be inserted at the first indication of an attack, and the patient should then lie down for an hour or so until the medicine takes effect.

Ergodryl. These capsules contain the same ingredients as Cafergot tablets with the addition of diphenhydramine (Benadryl), an antihistamine, and are used in the same way as Cafergot tablets.

Migral and Migril. These contain two milligrams of ergotamine tartrate, as well as caffeine and cyclizine as an antiemetic. Because the active agent is double the dose of that in Cafergot and Wigraine, it is advisable to take only one tablet at the onset of an attack, which may be repeated in one-half to one hour if required.

Some 70 percent of patients find that their attacks subside rapidly with adequate dosage of ergotamine tartrate medication if taken early enough. It is recommended that one not take ergotamine during pregnancy because it may cause mild contractions of the uterus, although I have not known its use during pregnancy to lead to miscarriage or cause other adverse effects. Indeed, if it were effective as an abortifacient, it would enjoy considerably greater sales than it does as a remedy for migraine. All of these preparations are best held in reserve for the acute attack and should not be taken regularly each day. If the frequency of attack increases, other measures must be taken, which are detailed below.

For those patients who cannot tolerate ergotamine or do not respond to its use, one of the range of nonsteroidal anti-inflammatory drugs can be tried. These drugs, such as naproxen (Naprosyn) or the fenemates, were introduced for the treatment of joint pains, but are effective in some patients with migraine. They may irritate the stomach, so it is best to take them with milk or something to eat. Isometheptene mucate has also been reported to abort migraine attacks (available in the U.S. in combination with caffeine and acetaminophen as Migralam or with acetaminophen and a sedative as Midrin).

Preventing Migraine

It is hoped that attention to psychological factors, elimination of precipitating causes, and relaxation exercises will help reduce the frequency and severity of migraine, and that the attacks will be abbreviated by the use of ergotamine preparations. However, the fact is that there are some people whose attacks will continue unabated in spite of these measures. And there are an unfortunate few whose attacks increase in frequency until they occur almost daily.

It is important to search for a cause for the increasing intensity of migraine. Among possible causes are use of the contraceptive pill, an increase in blood pressure, or the abuse of ergotamine preparations. The term "abuse" here means that the patient is taking these tablets every day in anticipation of a headache, whether or not one is developing. This habit may lead to a rebound headache as the vessels dilate when the effect of ergotamine wears off. Under these circumstances the doctor may recommend a week in the hospital so that the cycle can be broken. Often if a migraine sufferer can enjoy a short spell isolated from the responsibilities of everyday life while being regimented by the protective hospital routine, he or she can be freed of migraine and may be able permanently to alter the old pattern. The other possible cause to consider is the onset of a depressive state, which may require treatment with antidepressant tablets as well as psychological support.

A number of medications have proven valuable in reducing the frequency of migraine attacks when taken daily as a preventive measure. The agents usually employed first are known as beta blockers, because they block the beta receptors on which adrenaline works in the nervous system as well as on blood vessels. The beta blockers effective against migraine are propranolol (Inderal), atenolol (Tenormin), timolol (Blocadren), and metoprolol (Lopressor). The most commonly used is propranolol, which is marketed as 10-, 20-, 40-, 60-, 80-, and 90-milligram tablets. I usually start with 10 or 20 milligrams twice daily to ensure that it is well tolerated, slowly increasing the dosage until the headaches cease or a full beta-blocking dose is achieved. This may require a total dose of 240 to 320 milligrams each day. With full dosage, the pulse rate is slow and blood pressure drops when the person stands up, so dizziness may be a side effect. Some people may also be troubled by vivid dreams. Treatment may continue for a year or more.

The next line of defense involves the antiserotonin substances. These agents block the direct effect of serotonin on the blood vessels, where it is believed to be responsible for constricting the smaller arteries and their branches and for sensitizing the vessels to cause pain. One of these agents, methysergide, also increases the effect of any circulating substance that maintains tone in the larger arteries. Thus, it has a twofold action in preventing migraine.

Methysergide (Sansert, Deseril) is among the most efficient of all prophylactic agents for migraine. About one-third of all those who take it for the first time experience aching of the arms or legs, indigestion, or other odd symptoms for the first few days. Most of these symptoms disappear quite rapidly, but there remain some 10 percent of patients who cannot tolerate it. Of the other 90 percent, the majority either lose their headaches entirely or experience at least a 50 percent reduction in headache frequency. If ergotamine preparations have to be used to treat attacks that occur in spite of methysergide, they are usually more effective in getting rid of the headache than they were before. It is recommended that dosage start with one tablet three times daily, and I would suggest that on the first occasion a tablet be cut in half and taken as a test dose to ensure that it will be tolerated. You must be guided by your doctor as to the maximum dose allowed. Once improvement of the headache is established, the dose can be reduced to the minimum necessary to keep the attacks under control. Sometimes only one or two tablets each night will be sufficient to maintain improvement.

In the early days of methysergide treatment, when large doses were given continuously, some patients developed abdominal or chest pain caused by the excessive growth of fibrous tissue. Although this naturally gave rise to concern, these effects could be reversed by stopping treatment. Nowadays it is recommended that the pills be stopped altogether for one month out of every four to prevent the development of fibrotic side effects. Occasionally treatment may cause little veins in the cheeks and nose to become more prominent, but this is uncommon. The appetite may increase and some patients gain weight when taking methysergide, but this applies to many effective migraine remedies. If several vomiting days are replaced by several eating days each week, it is hard to avoid the tendency to gain weight—except by a general reduction of food intake spread over the whole week. Like the ergotamine preparations, methysergide may occasionally cause whiteness and numbness of the fingers or signs of constriction of vessels elsewhere. If so, this should be discussed at once with your doctor. The treatment may have to be stopped or used in combination with other tablets that block this excessive constrictor action, such as hydergine.

Other antiserotonin agents, such as pizotifen, pizotylene (Sandomigran), or cyproheptadine are also useful in preventing migraine in the daily dose of three or more tablets, best taken at night, as they may cause drowsiness. They may also stimulate the appetite so that weight-watching is necessary, but this is a small price to pay for freedom from headache. Loss of hair is a side effect often quoted as a disadvantage of the antiserotonin agents. With all the preparations we have tried, whether they be antiserotonin agents or not, periodic hair loss has been noted by 1 percent of patients. It seems probable that at any one time 1 percent of the female population is undergoing a "molting season." The hair may become a little thin, but in my experience it has always grown back again normally, whether or not the pills are continued.

A new group of antiserotonin agents has been developed to block the pain-producing effect of serotonin on blood vessels. Several of these have shown positive results in preliminary tests.

Recently, drugs have been used to stop the constriction of blood vessels by preventing the use of calcium necessary for this reaction. These are termed calcium channel blockers. Members of the group studied for the prevention of migraine include verapamil, nefedipine, nimodipine, and flunarazine. It is a little too early yet to say what part they will come to play in routine management. Anti-inflammatory drugs such as naproxen are beneficial in reducing the frequency of attacks in some people. Other agents, such as clonidine (Catapres), have proved disappointing. The antidepressant substance amitriptyline can be very helpful and is discussed in detail in chapter 8.

Finally, the group of drugs known as the monoamine oxidase (MAO) inhibitors have also been used with success in treating migraine (6). Because they require some restriction of diet, including the elimination of cheese and red wine, they are not altogether popular, but they can be kept in reserve for the patient who has tried everything and still continues to suffer from migraine. Foods that should not be eaten while taking MAO inhibitors, such as phenelzine (Nardil), include meat extracts, broad beans, pickled herring, and chicken livers, as well as cheese and red wines. No other medication should be taken at the same time without discussing it with your doctor.

What of the Future?

There is no one sure cure for migraine. Work is continuing in laboratories in many parts of the world. Scientists are studying the blood vessels, their reactions to various chemical substances and to stimulation of their nerve supply, and the effects of pharmaceutical agents directly on the nervous system. Others are examining the psychological basis of migraine and various physical factors that can affect the mind and, through it, the body. There is certainly great hope that in the future migraine can be removed from the list of scourges which make life unhappy for so many people. In the meantime much can be done with the tools we already possess, but it requires a conscientious and sustained effort by both patient and doctor.

8

PERHAPS
I HAVE TENSION
HEADACHE

Defining Tension Headache

If you have not recognized your symptoms in the chapters on
migraine, and if your headaches are not accompanied by visual
disturbance or vomiting, then you may have tension headache.
Tension headache may be defined as a constant tight, heavy,
or pressing sensation on or around the head, commonly affecting both sides of the head or neck simultaneously. In other
words, tension headache is a chronic headache without any
features of migraine. A number of neurologists and psychologists have tried without success to isolate combinations of characteristics that define common migraine and tension headache
as separate entities (32). The most reliable features for the
diagnosis of migraine are the episodic nature and relative brevity
of the attacks. Patients who have both types of headache distinguish between them on the grounds of severity and associated
symptoms, but this does not tell us whether they are basically
different disorders or different degrees of severity of the same
disorder.

We can distinguish between acute tension headache, coming
only at times of considerable stress or anxiety, and chronic
tension headache, which is present more or less all the time, "all
day and every day."

Clinical Features

Age and Sex Distribution

As with migraine, tension headache affects women two or three times more often than men. It may come on at any age (see Figure 8.1). About 15 percent of patients are under the age of ten years, and some patients are fifty years of age or over

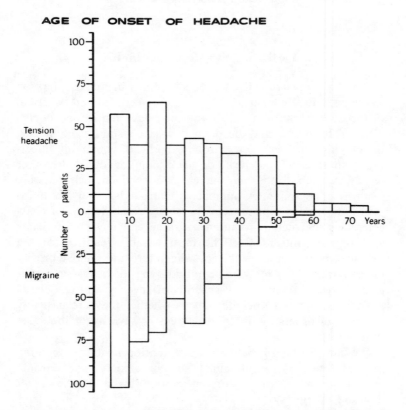

8.1 *The age of onset for tension headache as compared with migraine. These data are taken from a study conducted in our own clinic, a different control group from those analyzed in Figure 5.2 (68).*

when the headaches begin (68). Figure 8.1 shows a comparison of the age of onset of patients with tension and migraine headaches who attended one of our clinics.

Family History

Forty percent of patients with tension headache have a close relative with some form of chronic headache, but only 18 percent have a family history of migraine, about the same figure as in the general population.

Type of Headache

Tension headache affects both sides of the head in 90 percent of patients, in contrast to migraine, where in two-thirds of sufferers the headache is limited to one side of the head. The pain is usually dull and persistent and is felt as a pressure on top of the head or a band around it; some patients also experience jabs of sudden pain in the head (ice-pick pains) like their migrainous counterparts. Many people with tension headaches are liable to a periodic upsurge of pain like a miniature migraine, which is called tension-vascular headache for lack of a better term. Ten percent or more have definite migraine headaches superimposed on the daily background of discomfort. About half the patients have a headache every day of their lives, and this unfortunate state may persist for ten to thirty years, or possibly throughout their lifetime (see Figure 8.2).

Associated Features

Tension headache is often accompanied by a sense of depression or symptoms of anxiety. Patients may feel that life is joyless and that they are simply existing from day to day. They may have withdrawn from their previous social contacts and lost interest in their everyday routine, their work, and their hobbies. One common symptom of anxiety is hyperventilation. Without realizing it, the patient may take deep, sighing breaths at intervals throughout the day, which causes a constant feeling of lightheadedness, giddiness, or unsteadiness. Air may be swallowed as each deep breath is taken so that the stomach fills with

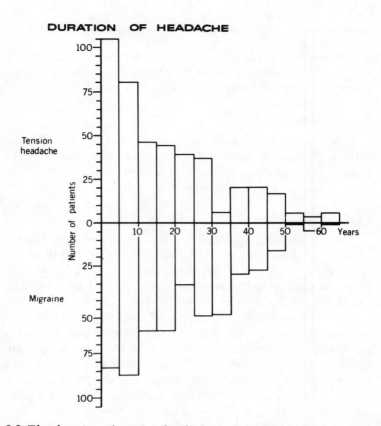

8.2 *The duration of tension headache and migraine as of the time patients were first seen in our neurological clinic.*

air and becomes bloated, the abdomen becomes tense and painful, and the patient feels the need to belch or pass wind frequently.

Some tense people are subject to an ache in their back or over the left side of their chest, as well as in the head. Others may also suffer from indigestion and nausea. There is often an aversion to the glare of sunlight, which causes the patient to wear dark glasses every day, regardless of whether it is sunny. Others may have sweaty palms. Tense people are often jaw-clenchers and may grind their teeth from side to side at night. Sideways jaw movement may be so severe as to cause soreness or bruising inside the mouth. Psychologists have considered this to be an atavistic trait, like an animal sharpening its fangs before a battle. In any event, it probably does represent repressed aggression.

Precipitating Factors

Some acute forms of tension headache are brought on by excessive muscle contraction, such as frowning or jaw-clenching. The astute observer may feel the forehead or jaw aching after a tense interview and realize that muscles have been working overtime. If there is an imbalance of the bite, often caused by teeth missing on one side of the jaw, strain is thrown onto the hinge joint of the jaw on one side of the mouth; pain is felt in front of the ear, radiating forward over the head, and the jaw muscles ache. Some patients who are subject to a pain or clicking in the neck hold their necks rigidly, with the result that the neck aches and pain spreads upward to the back of the head. Eyestrain can cause a tension headache because of frowning and squinting in an attempt to see clearly.

Tension headaches are usually made worse by stress, noise, or bright lights.

Relieving Factors

A pure tension headache may be eased by drinking alcohol or by smoking marijuana, but if there is a vascular component to the headache these activities make the headache more severe and throbbing in quality. Analgesics such as aspirin may relieve the headache for a period of hours, but patients who take increasing quantities of these substances each day run the risk of future kidney disease if this practice is continued over many years.

The Cause of Tension Headache

Personality and Psychological Factors

In the early stages, each headache usually has an identifiable cause, but if the headaches become progressively more frequent, it becomes harder to distinguish any external event that can be held responsible. Patients with chronic headache, like those suffering from other kinds of chronic pain, often deny that there is any real problem or worry in their lives. Is there some psychological factor in their constitution that makes them react unfavorably to the usual social, economic, or intellectual demands of life? There is an association between chronic tension headache and other illnesses commonly thought to be psychosomatic, such as duodenal ulcer and nervous diarrhea, but psychological tests show no startling differences in personality from the general population. However, there is a tendency to dwell on or embellish symptoms and to claim a number of additional disabilities, usually vaguely described. Anxiety and depression are present in almost all patients with chronic tension headache, compared with only about half those who suffer from migraine.

Muscle Contraction

It used to be thought that tension headache was caused by constant overcontraction of neck, jaw, and scalp muscles, possibly in conjunction with spasm of blood vessels supplying those muscles with oxygen. The muscles were thus overworked and underpaid. While this may apply in an acute tension state, it does not seem to be the case with chronic daily headaches. Careful studies have not shown any difference in the degree of muscle contraction in chronic tension-headache patients and headache-free subjects (75). Muscle contraction may not be essential for the development of tension headache, but it may play a part in prolonging and increasing its severity.

Vascular Factors

It has been shown earlier in this book that pain from blood vessels can be responsible for headache, particularly in migraine, and that blood flow in the scalp vessels often increases at that time. There must be some vascular component in tension headache, for on occasion the pain may become more severe and throb with the pulse, and blood flow then increases to the muscles. While substances that dilate blood vessels, such as alcohol, may help some patients with tension headache, they make the pain more severe in others. The infusion of histamine, a potent dilator agent, into the veins produces a pulsating headache in half the patients with tension headache and in almost all patients with migraine, whereas it has little effect on headache-free subjects given the same dose (58). It looks as though tension headache occupies an intermediate position in the spectrum of vascular headache, which ranges from head-ache freedom on one end to severe migraine headache at the other.

Neurotransmitters

The role of serotonin in migraine was discussed earlier. At the onset of migraine, blood platelets clump together and release their content of serotonin. The serotonin level rises and then drops below normal as it is adsorbed to blood vessels or destroyed in the body (5). In 1981 a group of research workers in Germany reported that the serotonin content of the blood was significantly lower in patients with tension headache than in headache-free subjects (95). Michael Anthony has recently confirmed this important observation in our laboratory. He found that the serotonin content (measured in billionths of a gram contained in a billion blood platelets) averaged 414 in twenty normal subjects, but only 276 in thirty patients with chronic tension headache. This suggests that chronic tension headache is a low-serotonin syndrome. It is quite possible that changes in the blood mirror changes in the nervous system. It will be recalled that serotonin plays an important part in the body's pain-control system (Figures 2.2 and 2.3 in chapter 2). If serotonin leaks out of this system, pain control is diminished and spontaneous aching may be felt in the head and other parts of the body as well. Serotonin also plays a part in registering emotion in the brain, and depletion of serotonin can cause de-pression. Perhaps tension headache and depression often occur in tandem because of this common factor.

Psychological Management

Chronic tension headache is a condition in which anxiety, depression, and dull, constant pain wax and wane together. For the reasons given above it cannot be attributed solely to emotional disturbance or failure to relax. Nevertheless, the attainment of a calm, relaxed state is an important step in getting rid of the headache and in some people may even obviate the need for medication.

It is important for sufferers to be reassured that they do not have a cerebral tumor or other structural abnormality that warrants surgery or other dramatic intervention. The problem should be discussed in realistic terms, and all potential forms of treatment weighed.

Some patients benefit from a discussion with their doctor of immediate or long-standing problems, without the need for formal psychotherapy. Expressing long-repressed feelings may aid in the treatment of headache. Many such anxieties are of sexual origin—possibly taking the form of fears about masturbation, guilt about premarital intercourse or later infidelity, anxiety about the possibility of venereal disease being acquired in the past (almost invariably groundless), or previously unvoiced feelings of homosexuality, especially with the present worry over AIDS as a potential consequence for the practicing homosexual. It took a number of interviews before a middle-aged man confessed that his life had been tarnished by a long-standing belief that masturbation in adolescence had been responsible for his undersized penis. He had always avoided using public dressing rooms because of the fear that other men would notice the size of his penis and associate it with his clandestine masturbation. The one person in whom he had confided in all these years provided no reassurance. When he was finally assured that masturbation was almost universal among adolescent boys, that the size of his penis was well within the normal range, and that there was no possible connection between the two, his whole attitude changed. His headache disappeared as though a cloud had been lifted, and he said, "Why couldn't I have been told this thirty years ago?" The reassurance that many experiences are quite normal can bring great relief to someone who has always regarded his or her particular problem as unique. Sexual counseling by a physician or psychiatrist skilled in this field can be of enormous assistance, particularly for specific problems such as impotence and premature ejaculation in men and frigidity in women.

Advice may also be required about the handling of everyday life situations. The following simple rules are taken from *Psychosomatic Medicine* by Edward Weiss and O. Spurgeon English of Philadelphia (113):

1. This is not a perfect world. Families and friends, too, have their failings. Perfection is rarely attained, so be satisfied with less.
2. Tolerance makes understanding the other fellow easier. It sets an attainable standard.
3. Do not be a slave to the clock. Work at your own pace. Do as much as you can. Trying to meet too many deadlines only creates tension.
4. You cannot please everybody, so stop trying. Popularity comes by giving your friends and family a chance to love you for yourself, not for your best performance.
5. Be efficient, yes, but not to the extent that perfection becomes a burden.
6. Speak up if you want to. You cannot please everybody, and honesty and directness break down barriers and make friendships easier.
7. Approve of yourself. You are as good as the next fellow.
8. Stop being so critical of your negative feelings. Everyone is ambivalent at times, so do not worry so much about loving and hating.
9. Stop feeling so guilty. We are all human beings, and we all make errors. Give a little and you will get a lot—maybe even a reduction of the pain in your head.

Explanation and advice about one's style of life and its associated problems may be all that is required. However, some patients may benefit from formal psychotherapy, and those patients with severe depression or thought disorders are best referred to a psychiatrist as soon as this is recognized.

Physical Management

There are many patients whose problems are either in-apparent or insoluble. Some of them say that they have not a care in the world apart from their headache, while others admit to persisting symptoms of anxiety and depression. In either case, it is important to establish a satisfactory pattern of living, with regular daily exercise and the right balance of work and leisure time. A little joy and laughter helps too. The aim is to achieve a state of mental and physical relaxation. Although excessive muscle contraction is no longer considered the most important factor in tension headache, gaining control over one's muscles is still the key to physical comfort and diminishes the sense of tension and anxiety. The concept is not new, but it is now being used more frequently in the management of headache problems, with or without biofeedback, as discussed in chapter 7 (11, 112).

Dr. Edmund Jacobsen of Chicago made notable early contributions to the subject, and there have since been other books that are also useful reading for anyone subject to tension headache (54). Based on the principles of these authors, a simple series of relaxation exercises for patients is suggested. The only basic difference between my recommendations and those of others is my emphasis on a positive attempt to relax, to "switch off" the muscle mechanisms. Ideally, the initial sessions should take place in the presence of an instructor who can ensure that the correct sequence is being carried out and that the subject is indeed relaxing correctly.

Are You Able to Relax?

The blood vessels and nerve fibers of the scalp lie in muscle. Place your fingers on each temple and clench your jaw. You will feel the temporal muscle swell as it contracts. Let the jaw go loose and the muscle becomes flat again. Many people contract these muscles all day without realizing it, so they are working continuously. This sets up a constant dull ache in the temples. Do you feel the jaw muscles aching at the end of the day, or after an unpleasant or difficult conversation, or after an argument? Do you feel an ache in one or both temples at these times, or do you wake up with a headache in this area?

Just as chronic jaw-clenching is a common cause of aching in the temples, chronic frowning is a common cause of pain in the forehead. Do others say to you that you frown a lot or look worried most of the time? This can be an indication that you are using your scalp muscles without being aware of it. Pain in the neck can also result from muscle contraction. Some people walk about holding their necks stiffly, as though they were solid blocks of wood. Overcontraction of muscle is a faulty habit that develops over the years and often starts in childhood. It may be associated with mental tension and anxiety but may also have become an automatic reaction that continues even when there are no problems.

The most natural form of treatment is training the muscles of the body to relax. The first step is to realize that you are not as relaxed as you think you are.

Try these simple tests:

1. Sit in a chair and lean back. Ask someone to lift your arm in the air into a comfortable position as though it were resting on the side of an armchair. Take your time and relax completely. Then ask your friend to take away his or her hands, which have been supporting your arm. When the supporting hands are taken away, what does your arm do?

   If it flops lifelessly downward, you are indeed relaxed. If it stays in the air, or you move it slowly downward, you are not relaxed (see Figure 8.3a, b). Your muscles are contracting continuously *without your realizing it.*

2. Lie on a bed or couch with your head on a pillow and try to relax completely. When you consider that you have achieved this, ask your associate to pull the pillow away from under your head.

   Does your head drop limply onto the bed? Or does it stay poised in midair as though the pillow were still there?

   If you are still holding your head in the air above an invisible pillow, your muscles are contracting *without your realizing it* (see Figure 8.3c, d).

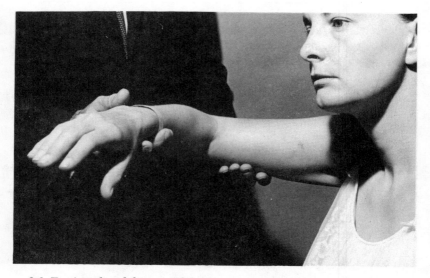

8.3 *Testing the ability to relax. (a.) The patient is instructed to let her arm muscles go loose in the examiner's hand, as though she were relaxing in an armchair.*

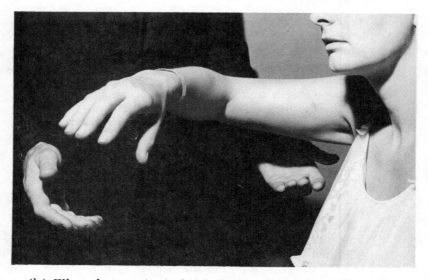

(b.) When the examiner's hands are removed, the patient's arm remains in the same position, which indicates that she is not relaxed.

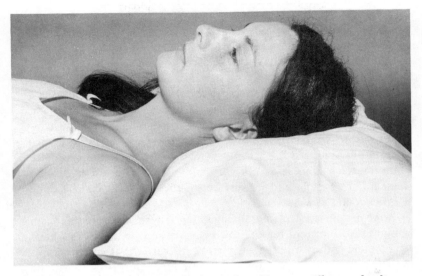

(c.) The patient is told to lie back comfortably on a pillow and relax her neck muscles.

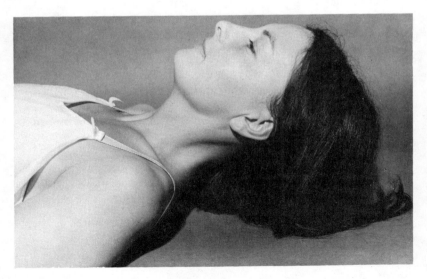

(d.) When the pillow is removed, her head remains in a rigid, contracted position, rather than flopping back as it would in a relaxed state.

Once you have acknowledged that excessive muscle contraction is playing a part in the aching of your head or neck, and that you do not really know whether the muscles are contracting or not, you are ready to start relaxation exercises.

Paradoxically, you cannot relax about relaxing. It is not a passive process. It is no use saying to someone, "Relax," and imagining that he can do it without further thought. You cannot say to yourself, "Relax," and then do it, unless you have carefully practiced the art of "switching off" the nerve supply to the muscles. This is a voluntary action as deliberate as turning off a light switch, and it must be practiced until it can be done quickly and at will.

At first it is necessary to set aside at least ten minutes each night and morning for the exercises. It is a great help to have someone with you in the early stages to verify that you are completely relaxed when you think you are. This person will be referred to below as the "assistant." It is obviously a great advantage if the assistant can be a trained physiotherapist or occupational therapist, but this is not always practicable. A well-motivated companion can be of enormous value in ensuring that the exercises are performed conscientiously and that relaxation is practiced until it becomes second nature.

The Sequence of Relaxation Exercises

Lie down on a firm surface such as a carpeted floor. A bed with an inner-spring mattress will do, but not one with a soft, sagging mattress. A pillow can be used to support the head at first but may be discarded later as relaxation becomes easier. For the first few sessions a short-sleeved shirt and shorts should be worn so that muscle contraction can be seen as well as felt. Lie on your back with legs slightly separated and arms comfortably flexed at the elbows so that they are by the sides of your trunk, with the hands resting on the body. Various muscles will be contracted and relaxed in turn.

1. *Legs.* Contract the leg muscles so that the legs become rigid. The muscles will stand out as they contract. Concen-

trate on the sensation of muscle contraction and the feeling of tension in the legs. Then, suddenly and deliberately, "switch off the power supply" so that the muscles become limp. Concentrate on whether any sensation is now coming from the muscles. Are they completely relaxed? At this point it is helpful for an assistant to put a hand behind the subject's knees and lift them up sharply to see whether the leg is completely floppy and if the muscles will contract again as soon as the limb is moved passively. If they are not completely relaxed or if they contract again when the limb is touched or moved, the sequence should be repeated. Many people only half relax on the first few attempts. This can be detected by closely watching the muscles. After the first relaxation exercise, the muscles are not as prominent as they were initially, but there may be some contraction remaining. Try again to "switch off," and this second attempt may be rewarded by the muscle becoming completely flaccid. The assistant may then bend the legs at the knee, move them about, or roll them backward and forward with the feet flailing like a rag doll. This sequence may be completed by lifting one leg, letting it drop downward like an inanimate object, and then doing the same with the other.

2. *Arms.* Brace the arms so that the elbows are forced downward on the couch (or on the assistant's hand if he or she is checking the degree of relaxation). Hold the arms rigid and then stop the muscle contraction suddenly so that the arms become limp and lifeless. The assistant should then be able to bounce the elbow up and down without any resistance being offered. This sequence should be repeated until the subject is aware of both the sensation of muscle contraction and the contrast with the feeling of relaxation. The assistant should also be satisfied that the arm has become flaccid.

3. *Neck.* Lift the head from the pillow and then allow it to drop backward. The assistant may provide resistance by pressing on the forehead until the subject feels the contraction of the muscles in the front of the neck. When the head is dropped backward, the assistant can rock it gently to and fro to make certain that there is no residual activity in the muscles. Now push the head backward into the pillow and

register the sensation of contraction of the muscles in the back of the neck. Stop the contraction suddenly so that the assistant may rotate the head freely on the neck. Repeat this until relaxation is satisfactory.

4. *Forehead.* Frown upward so that the brow is furrowed. If there is difficulty in doing this, look upward as far as the eyes will move until the forehead becomes creased. Again, feel the sensation of tension in the muscles, then close the eyes and let the forehead muscles relax. The assistant can detect the presence or absence of contraction by seeing whether the skin of the forehead moves freely with his or her hand.

5. *Eyes.* Screw the eyes up tightly and become aware of the sensation of tension, then relax the muscles and lie with the eyes closed lightly. Make sure that there is no trembling or flickering of the closed eyelids and that the eye muscles feel entirely relaxed.

6. *Jaw.* Clench the jaw firmly and concentrate on feeling the sense of tightness in the temples as well as in the jaw itself. Then switch off and let the jaw loll open. Push the jaw open, perhaps against the pressure of the assistant's hand, then relax completely. Move the jaw sideways to the right as far as it will go and experience the sensation felt in the jaw and temple before relaxing. Then do the same to the left. Complete the sequence by clenching the jaw firmly again, and let the jaw drop open loosely. The assistant should then be able to hold the tip of the jaw with his or her fingers and waggle the jaw up and down rapidly without any opposition from the jaw muscles (see Figure 8.4).

This is the hardest of all relaxation exercises, and you must not be disappointed if you are unsuccessful on the first attempt. It may require repeated practice to get the jaw muscles to cease all activity so that the jaw may be moved easily by the assistant. It is most important that you persevere and master the switching-off process, for over-contraction of jaw muscles is the most common factor in tension headache.

7. *Whole body relaxation.* Once you are able to relax the legs, arms, neck, forehead, eye, and jaw muscles in that order, lie for five minutes with all muscles relaxed. When

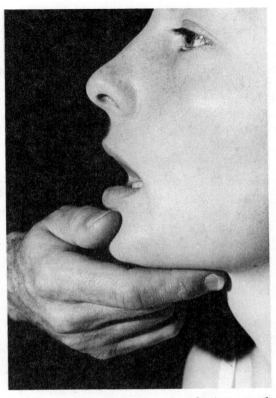

8.4 *Relaxing the jaw. The ability to relax the jaw muscles can be tested by an examiner who moves the jaw rapidly up and down. In most patients with tension headache, the jaw is held rigidly, so that the head and jaw move together.*

you have achieved total relaxation, the process becomes negative rather than positive. In other words, you allow natural relaxation to continue rather than willing yourself to relax. At this stage, it is helpful to think of some beautiful and tranquil scene, to imagine yourself lying on a grassy bank on a warm summer's day with the drowsy sounds of summer in the background. Everyone has some particular sound he or she associates with peace and tranquility. It may be the rippling of a trout stream, the humming of bees, the song of birds, the sighing of wind in the trees, or distant music. Choose your own theme and your own mental picture and live in that scene for a few minutes. As you do so, feel the sensation of heaviness creep over your legs, trunk, and arms, then move up to your neck and head, eyes, and face. Feel the sense of freedom in your mind and head. This can become a permanent freedom if you train your muscles to obey at other times as well as they are responding at this moment.

After Relaxation Exercises Are Finished

The final and most important step is to carry the art of relaxation into your everyday life. On a typical day, watch the way you stand, sit, converse with people, write, type, or perform any other activity. Check that all the muscles not essential to the task of the moment are in a state of relaxation. You can handle any situation, irrespective of the degree of mental stress, without physical tension once you become accustomed to this routine. You actually perform more efficiently if you tackle any problem is an orderly fashion without excessive and useless muscle contraction. If you notice any warning sensations of tension in the scalp, jaw, or neck muscles, you must pause a moment to ensure that these muscles are "switched off" in the manner you have practiced. In this way you will finish the day feeling much fresher and will have much less chance of a headache ruining your day.

Keep Practicing

There is no point in performing the exercise routine religiously for a week and then forgetting the whole thing. If you do, the old habits of muscle contraction will assert themselves again. Keep practicing, stay relaxed, and help rid yourself of tension headache.

Medication

Some twenty years ago when we were just starting the systematic study of headache problems in our clinic and laboratory, Dr. Don Curran and I found that many patients continued to have tension headaches despite psychological counseling and relaxation therapy (67). We undertook a study of the effects of various medications in 280 patients with tension headache, 239 of whom were subject to daily headaches. Various pharmaceutical agents were prescribed for a month in turn and the response was assessed. Dummy (placebo) tablets were given to twenty of the patients for comparison, and six members of this group did improve. Agents that gave no better response than the placebo included a barbiturate, vasodilator drugs (to increase blood flow to face and scalp), methysergide (an effective antimigraine agent), and orphenadrine (used for the muscular rigidity of Parkinson's disease). The most effective medication proved to be the antidepressant amitriptyline, which benefited two-thirds of the patients, followed by another antidepressant, imipramine.

We then undertook a "double-blind" trial of amitriptyline in twenty-seven patients. The term "double-blind" means that neither the patient nor the doctor knows whether the patient is receiving the active medication or a placebo tablet until the trial ends, in order to remove any possibility of bias. At the end of the month patients switched from amitriptyline to the placebo or vice-versa. No patient responded to the placebo alone, twelve patients responded to amitriptyline alone, and three improved in both treatment periods. Since that trial, amitriptyline has been used as a standard method of treatment for chronic tension headaches in most parts of the world and is now used to suppress migraine attacks as well.

Because amitriptyline is an antidepressant, does that mean that all patients with chronic headaches are depressed? Not really. It has been pointed out that serotonin helps regulate the pain-control system as well as maintain a normal emotional state. The function of amitriptyline is to prevent the re-uptake of serotonin into nerve cells, thereby making more serotonin available as a neurotransmitter. Our own trial showed that amitriptyline worked just as well whether patients were depressed or not.

Amitriptyline (for which there are many trade names) is usually available as 10- and 25-milligram tablets. My own practice is initially to prescribe a small dose, say 10 or 12.5

milligrams, to be taken at bedtime in case it makes the recipient drowsy. This side effect is unpredictable. Some patients will feel dopey on a small dose and others will be alert after taking a large dose (six or more of the 25-milligram tablets each night), probably because the blood levels attained vary tenfold in individuals of similar weight given the same dose. I slowly increase the dose from one-half to one of the 25-milligram tablets, to two tablets, and finally to three tablets taken at night. In this way any drowsiness is usually dispelled by morning, and the next day the patient experiences only slight dryness of the mouth, indicating that a satisfactory blood level has been achieved. Trembling hands, blurred vision, and slowness in starting to pass urine are less common side effects. Amitriptyline can be highly successful for those patients who tolerate it well, diminishing or abolishing tension headache within two to ten days of starting treatment. Medication should then be maintained for at least six months before the patient is weaned off it. For those patients subject to side effects, other antidepressant agents such as imipramine or tranquilizers such as chlordiazepoxide (Librium) or diazepam (Valium) can be used, although they are somewhat less effective.

For patients resistant to these medications, the monoamine oxidase (MAO) inhibitor phenelzine (Nardil) can be prescribed, as it prevents the breakdown of serotonin and noradrenaline in the body. This drug is also effective in treating migraine, but it must be used with caution, since certain foods and drugs must not be ingested by any patients treated with MAO inhibitors. These have been mentioned in chapter 7 but are worth repeating. Prohibited foods include cheese, meat extracts, broad beans, pickled herring, chicken livers, and packet soups (which are rich in tyramine, a monoamine that liberates noradrenaline in the body and can therefore cause a dangerous increase in blood pressure because monoamines can no longer be broken down in the body). Nose drops, weight-reducing pills, or any tablets for colds or sinusitis must not be used, because these all contain monoamines. Ordinary analgesics or migraine tablets can be taken, but no injections should be given without the knowledge and supervision of the prescribing doctor.

Conclusions

I would like to be able to conclude by saying that a healthy life-style combined with mental and physical relaxation is enough to prevent tension headache. This is true sometimes, but not always. Some patients appear to have a deficiency of monoamines in their nervous system, which requires medication to adjust. Fortunately, the combination of psychological and pharmaceutical approaches will abolish or ease this depressing malady in the majority of patients.

9

I WOULD CERTAINLY KNOW IF I HAVE CLUSTER HEADACHE

Why?

Because cluster headache is a distinctive pain syndrome that can be recognized by the fact that it recurs in bouts, it regularly appears at a certain hour of the day or night, and it is associated with certain consistent features, such as redness and watering of the eye on the same side of the face as the site of pain. Unlike migraine and tension headache, cluster headache affects men much more often than women.

Definition

Cluster headache is a severe, one-sided head or facial pain, usually centered on one eye, that lasts for minutes or hours and recurs one or more times in a twenty-four-hour period (59). When the pain is severe, the eye on the affected side becomes red and waters, the eyelid may droop, and the nostril on the same side becomes blocked or runs. The term "cluster headache" derives from the tendency for the pain to recur in bouts lasting either weeks or months, after which it disappears completely for months or years. This recurring pattern of pain is found in 80 percent of patients and is known as episodic cluster headache.

In about 20 percent of patients there are no remissions from the pain. In this condition, the pains recur regularly, either on a daily basis or several times each week for a year or more without any break. This form is therefore called chronic cluster headache.

Finally, there is a rare variant in which the pains are shorter in duration but recur six or more times per day—up to twenty or so attacks each day. This has been given the name chronic paroxysmal hemicrania (CPH) (103).

Cluster headache is often confused with trigeminal neuralgia (tic douloureux) because of the severity of the pain, but unlike tic, which strikes with stabs as brief as a lightning flash, the pains in cluster headache last for ten minutes or more at a time. It is also confused with migraine, hence the alternative term "migrainous neuralgia," which is still favored in Britain.

A Historical Note

The condition was first described in 1840 by Moritz H. Romberg, then professor of medicine at the University of Berlin, a fact forgotten by English-speaking authors, who usually attribute its discovery to Dr. Wilfred Harris of London in 1926 (96, 49). Romberg used the term "ciliary neuralgia," because "ciliary" means related to the eyes or the eyelashes, and the pain of cluster headache usually centers around the eye. He wrote: "The pupil is contracted. The pain not unfrequently extends over the head and face. The eye generally weeps and becomes red. The symptoms occur in paroxyms, of a uniform or irregular character, and isolated or combined with facial neuralgia and hemicrania." Romberg considered that it might be caused by tuberculosis of the glands in the neck, a common disease of that time. He also thought it could be "brought on by discharges, especially seminal emissions," and "the development of puberty," among a long list otherwise irrelevant. The possible causes quoted are relevant, however, because cluster headache frequently begins in teenage boys, although the cause of the relationship remains obscure.

The condition was rediscovered and renamed in the 1930s by Dr. B. T. Horton, a physician at the Mayo Clinic, Rochester, Minnesota (52). Dr. Horton and his colleagues believed cluster headache was caused by the release of histamine, gave it the name histaminic cephalgia, and treated it by histamine desensitization. In our laboratories, Dr. Michael Anthony has now shown that histamine is indeed released during the pain of cluster headache, but whether it plays any part in its causation remains uncertain (7).

The term in current use, cluster headache, was coined by Dr. Charles Kunkle and his colleagues in 1954 (60).

A Unique Headache Pattern

Once encountered, the distinct pain of cluster headache is unlikely to be confused with anything else. The pain is invariably one-sided and usually sticks to the same side of the head, although there have been instances of it changing from one side to another in the middle of a bout. It is felt deeply behind one eye in 60 percent of patients, but it commonly radiates to the forehead, temple, cheek, and upper gum on the same side of the face (see Figure 9.1). The nostril on that side may ache and burn and usually is blocked or runs with fluid. Sometimes the palate may also be involved, and aching may spread to the lower gum, jaw, ear, or even the neck.

Usually, the pain of cluster headache is extraordinarily severe once the bout is established. The patient may leap up and stride back and forth while holding a hand over the eye. More temperate descriptions of the pain employ adjectives like burning, boring, piercing, tearing, and screwing. The pain usually comes on suddenly, lasts from ten minutes to several hours, and then dies away. It usually returns two or three times in the twenty-four-hour period, and commonly awakens the patient from sleep. The pain will often recur at the same time every day and night for a period of two to eight weeks and occasionally longer (see Figure 9.2). It then mercifully remits, only to recur months or years later. The average frequency in our patients was one bout per year, but many had two each year, and an unfortunate few suffered three or four bouts (see Figure 9.3) (65). At the other end of the scale, some patients had intervals of freedom of three to four years between bouts.

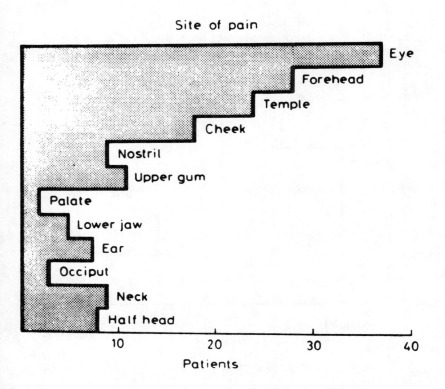

Site of pain

9.1 *The pain of cluster headache. Horizontal bars indicate the number of patients experiencing pain in each particular site. Sixty patients participated in this study (65).*

Age and Sex Distribution

The disorder usually develops between the ages of ten and thirty, although we have known patients to experience it for the first time even in old age (see Figure 9.4). In the episodic and chronic forms, 85 percent of those affected are male. In the uncommon variation, CPH, in which there are many brief attacks each day, women are affected more than men.

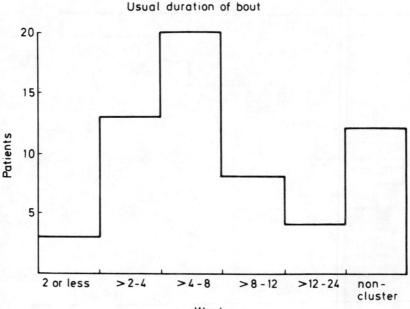

9.2 *The usual duration of each bout of cluster headaches measured in weeks.*

Some Curious Aspects

As the pain becomes severe, the eye on the affected side becomes bloodshot and may water. The eyelid droops and the pupil often constricts, indicating that the sympathetic nerve to the eye is no longer functioning on that side (see Figure 9.5). Vision may become blurred in the affected eye. The nostril becomes blocked or runs on one or both sides. The forehead may flush and sweat, and the patient sometimes feels slightly nauseated. The arteries may dilate on the side of the headache as they do in migraine, and the scalp often feels tender to the touch. The eye may appear puffy, and little lumps may be felt inside the mouth, like hives.

During the period of a cluster headache, any substance that dilates blood vessels will promptly trigger an attack. Alcohol is

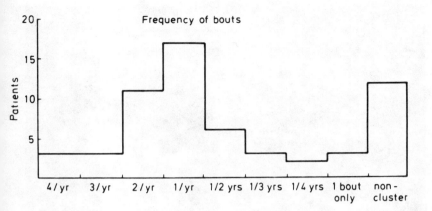

9.3 *The frequency of bouts of cluster headache in a study of 60 patients. The "non-cluster" column refers to those patients with no remissions (chronic cluster headache).*

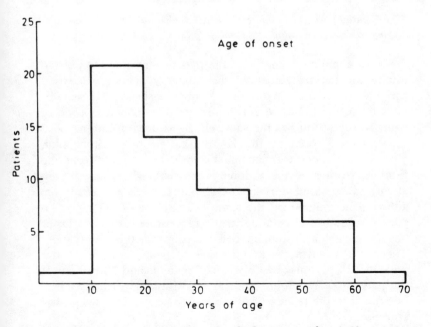

9.4 *The age of onset of cluster headache in a study of 60 patients (65).*

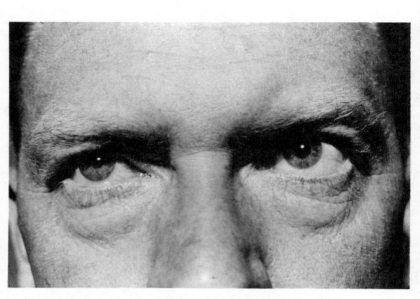

9.5 *A patient experiencing cluster headache, whose affected side displays a drooping eyelid and small pupil.*

the most common enemy, and the patient may have to abstain totally for the remainder of the bout. A patient who used carbon tetrachloride in his dry-cleaning business said that inhalation of the fumes would immediately set off an episode of pain. Nitroglycerin has the same effect, as does histamine.

Dr. Karl Ekbom of the Karolinska Hospital, Stockholm, reported a patient with angina pectoris (chest pain resulting from narrowing of the coronary arteries) whose chest pain almost disappeared during several bouts of cluster headache, although he maintained the same exercise load (36). A vasodilator substance circulating in the bloodstream during cluster headache, such as histamine, could account for this observation. There is also an increased incidence of peptic ulcer in cluster patients (14 percent of Ekbom's 105 patients and 20 percent of the patients of Dr. John Graham of Boston), which may well be related to the release of histamine, since it stimulates gastric secretion.

A family history of cluster headache is found in less than 5 percent of cases (59). Dr. John Graham of the Faulkner Hospital, Jamaica Plain, Boston, has drawn attention to the distinctive facial appearance of many patients subject to cluster headache—a furrowed, thick skin with a ruddy complexion (45).

Is This a Variation of Migraine?

There are certainly many similarities between the symptoms of migraine and of cluster headache, but the differences are even more striking. Cluster headache is much less common than migraine in the population, in a proportion of about one to twenty. Cluster headache affects males predominantly, while migraine is more common in women. Cluster headache rarely starts in childhood—one of our patients had a single, brief pain at the age of eight—while it is quite usual for migraine to start under the age of ten. It is possible for patients to suffer from both disorders. One patient of mine had the extraordinary and unpleasant experience of having a bout of cluster headache overlap with an increased frequency of migraine attacks, one affecting the left side of his head and the other the right. He was never in any doubt about the different characteristics of the two types of pain. Cluster headache is almost invariably unilateral, while migraine may spread to both sides of the head or be bilateral from the start. The focal neurological symptoms that are so often a part of the migraine attack—the flashing lights in front of the eyes, pins and needles, and other sensations—are extremely rare in cluster headache. Thermograms, measuring the heat loss from the head, show a warm spot in the temple in about one-third of migraine cases (Figure 6.2). This contrasts with cluster headache, where temperature increases in the orbit and the warm patch then spreads down the check or chin over the areas in which pain is experienced (see Figure 9.6a) (34).

Finally, the biochemical changes that have been found in our laboratory appear to demarcate the two conditions just as clearly as does the clinical pattern. Blood serotonin drops sharply in migraine but does not alter in cluster headache. Blood histamine elevates sharply in cluster headache, but in migraine a small increase becomes apparent only at the conclusion of an attack (7).

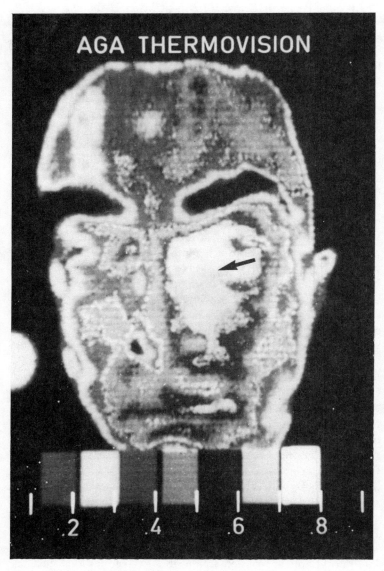

9.6 *(a.) Thermogram of the face taken during cluster headache. The white area over the patient's painful left eye, nostril, and cheek (arrowed) is about 1.8° Fahrenheit (1° Centigrade) warmer than the unaffected side.*

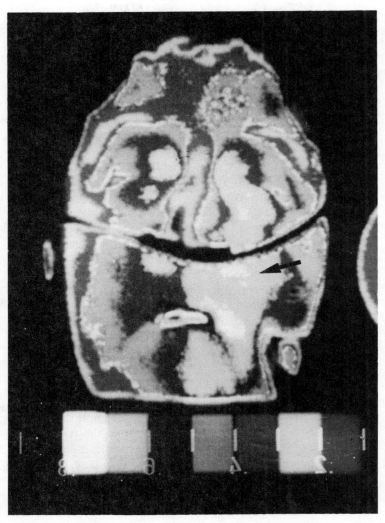

(b.) Thermogram taken after coagulation of the trigeminal ganglion. The white area (arrowed) shows that the eye, nostril, cheek, and chin are warmer on the operated side. Note the similarity with cluster headache in the distribution of the facial flush. The dark lines converging on the patient's nose are oxygen tubes.

The Cause of Cluster Headache

The Pain

During cluster headache, pain in some areas, such as the temples, can be relieved by pressure applied to that spot, but pain behind the eye remains static or becomes worse. Blood flow to the face and scalp increases during these painful episodes. This is particularly noticeable in the orbit, as pulsation of the eye and fluid pressure in the eye increase while the temperature of the whole orbit rises by 1.8 degrees Fahrenheit (1 degree Centigrade) or more in the majority of patients (21). The warm area then spreads over the parts of the face where the pain is felt (Figure 9.6a). It is unlikely that these vascular changes cause the pain, because the usual sequence of events is that the pain is well established before the increased skin temperature spreads over the painful areas.

For comparison, we have made some interesting observations on the facial flush seen in patients after thermocoagulation of the trigeminal ganglion, an operation to relieve the stabbing pains of trigeminal neuralgia (30). This procedure consists of inserting a probe under local anesthesia until it touches the trigeminal ganglion (Figure 2.2). The ganglion is then stimulated by electrical impulses so that the patient feels tingling in the face. The position of the probe is adjusted to cause tingling only over the area where the jabbing pain is commonly experienced, as in the cheeks or chin, for example. A general anesthetic is then injected into the arm while the temperature of the probe is increased in order to destroy the cells in the ganglion that convey pain sensation from that area. As this is being done, a flush appears over the affected part of the face, which can be recorded by thermography (see Figure 9.6b). It can be seen that the appearance of the flush in cluster headache and of the flush after the operation on the trigeminal nerve is remarkably similar. This brings up the possibility that the trigeminal pain pathways discharge spontaneously to cause cluster headache and that the changes in blood flow and temperature in the face are secondary to this, caused by a reflex through the nervous system or the release of substance P or VIP, as discussed in chapter 2. One patient of mine had both cluster headache and trigeminal neuralgia (the two conditions are sometimes associated). He was not completely unconscious when thermocoagulation started and said that the pain he experienced was exactly like that of his cluster headache.

The pain and the vascular changes of cluster headache are not always associated. In some patients the face does not flush, even though the pain is severe. On the other hand, there have been instances when patients on medication experienced watering of the eye and blockage of the nostril without pain developing. There must be two pathways involved. One is the pain-carrying trigeminal system and the other is the outgoing parasympathetic nerve that makes the blood vessels of the eye, nostril, and other parts of the face dilate. Both pathways can discharge independently, but one is usually linked with the other.

The Eye

Why does the eyelid droop and the pupil contract on the side of the headache? This is a sign that the sympathetic nerve to the eye is not working properly. The sympathetic nervous system prepares us for any emergency. If we are frightened or angry, the eye widens and the pupil dilates as part of our general state of alertness. If something goes wrong with the sympathetic nerves, the gap between the eyelids narrows and the pupil contracts (Figure 9.5). How could the sympathetic nerve be compromised on the affected side in cluster headache? There is a single report of an arteriogram being done while the pain was present. This showed that a localized part of the internal carotid artery leading up to the brain was narrow, indicating that the wall of the artery was swollen at that point. This could be relevant, for the sympathetic nerve forms a network around the internal carotid artery and would be compressed and put out of action if the wall were swollen. This theory fits quite well with the facts, since sweating on the forehead is caused by sympathetic nerves that run along the *external* carotid artery supplying blood to the face and scalp, and patients usually sweat normally or even excessively during the cluster pains. The sympathetic nerve to the eye must therefore be involved around the *internal* carotid artery after it has separated in its pathway from the fibers that control sweating. Why should the wall of the artery swell? The liberation of histamine could be responsible, causing a lump like the hives seen in the skin as a result of allergic reactions. It is also possible that the parasympathetic nerves, which cause dilatation of arteries supplying the face in cluster headache, could alter the small blood vessels in the wall of the carotid artery to cause a local swelling and knock out the sympathetic nerve on its travels.

The Neck

The neck often becomes painful and, as is also the case in migraine, there is often a tender spot felt at the base of the skull. Injecting this tender spot with a local anesthetic and a long-acting steroid will sometimes relieve the pain of cluster headache, at least temporarily. A syndrome like cluster headache has been reported after whiplash injury to the neck, and certain patients can bring on cluster pains by putting their necks in a certain position. It is probable that the inflow of impulses along the upper nerve roots in the neck can trigger off pain in the trigeminal system by the mechanism described in chapter 2 (Figure 2.1).

The Timing

The most fascinating aspect of cluster headache is its timing. There must be two internal clocks involved: one to start and stop the bout of headaches every year or so, and one to start and stop the pain once or more every twenty-four hours. As yet, we do not know the nature of these internal clocks, but they can be extraordinarily accurate. A patient of mine who frequently travels across Australia from Perth to Sydney (a 2,000-mile journey with a two-hour change in time zones) told me that his cluster headaches continued to wake him from sleep on Perth time until he adjusted his biological rhythms, when the headaches woke him at the same hour on Sydney time!

Treating Each Cluster as It Comes

There is no way known at present to abolish cluster headache permanently. There are, however, many nonmedical tricks that can be used to suppress the headaches and alleviate discomfort, as well as prescription drugs.

The Acute Attack

The most effective way to abolish the pain of cluster headache is to inhale 100 percent oxygen flowing at the rate of eight liters per minute through a resuscitation mask. This may sound impractical for home use, but it is relatively easy to install an oxygen cylinder, reduction valve, and mask in the home. First, the technique should be tried in a doctor's office or hospital to see if it works satisfactorily for that particular person. Four out of every five people find that the headache eases after about ten minutes of oxygen inhalation. If so, an oxygen cylinder at home or work may be the solution. Oxygen probably relieves the pain by constricting the blood vessels, and it may have other relevant actions on the central nervous system. (Since oxygen makes any flame burn more fiercely, cigarettes, matches, or any source of fire must be kept well away from the oxygen supply.)

Ergotamine preparations are not as useful for acute attacks of cluster as they are for migraine, because the episodes of cluster pain are shorter, and there is little time for ergotamine to be absorbed. If used, ergotamine is best given as an aerosol spray (pressure pack or Medihaler), which is absorbed rapidly from the lungs, or injected intramuscularly.

Recently a synthetic form of the hormone somatostatin has been given by infusion to ease the pain of cluster headache. This is of theoretical interest, as somatostatin blocks the release of substances P and VIP, which are thought to help cause pain and flushing.

Suppression of the Bout

Ergotamine can be used as a preventive measure by taking one or two tablets each night or twice daily, so that there is sufficient time for the ergotamine to be absorbed in order to stop the next episode. Ergotamine or dihydroergotamine (DHE) can also be injected once or twice daily at least one hour before the expected onset of the headache. Ergotamine is usually effective in the first or second bout of cluster headache but may lose its potency in subsequent bouts.

Methysergide (Deseril) is helpful in about 70 percent of patients, but it must be given in higher dosage than is necessary to prevent migraine. Since few bouts of cluster last longer than three months, there is little risk of any long-term side effect. Methysergide can give rise to adverse reactions, as mentioned in chapter 7, so a test done of one-half tablet is advisable before starting maintenance therapy three times a day. Propranolol (Inderal) and other drugs that are useful in migraine are not of much help in cluster headache.

The most consistently successful method of stopping a bout is a prescribed course of corticosteroids, such as prednisone, 60 to 75 milligrams per day for three days, with the daily dose slowly reduced thereafter. This stops the bout in three-quarters of patients. The dose is eventually reduced to the point where some headaches reappear, at which point the dose is adjusted up a notch and maintained at a suitable level to suppress the headaches until the bout ends. Thereafter, the daily dose is reduced gradually and then eliminated. If prednisone or other steroids have been taken for more than a week, the medication should never be stopped suddenly. Weaning off medication slowly allows the body's adrenal glands to start manufacturing their own brand of steroid to take over when the treatment ceases. Those patients with a past history of tuberculosis or severe mental disorder, among other conditions, should not be given steroid treatment.

Chronic Cluster Headache

When cluster headache persists for many months or even years without remission, corticosteroids cannot be used because of the hazard of long-term side effects. Ergotamine or methysergide may be useful for a while, but prolonged therapy is undesirable.

There are two forms of medical treatment that may help to keep chronic cluster headache under control. The first is lithium carbonate. This is administered as one tablet two or three times daily; a blood sample is taken at weekly intervals in order to adjust the dose so as to maintain an appropriate blood level. If the blood level is too high, patients may become shaky or confused. Use over a long period of time may occasionally cause kidney problems, and patients on lithium, or indeed any of the medications mentioned in this chapter, should remain under the close supervision of their doctor.

The second mode of attack is quite recent. In chapter 7, calcium-channel-blocking agents—such as verapamil, nefedepine, and nimodopine—were mentioned in the treatment of migraine. These prevent the constriction of blood vessels by stopping the uptake of calcium necessary for this reaction. The continued use of these agents for two months is said to settle down the chronic cluster headache in about 85 percent of patients. Recently, Dr. Michael Anthony of my department has been blocking the occipital nerves at the base of the skull with injections of a local anesthetic agent and a long-acting steroid. This often stops the chronic cluster cycle for days or weeks, but the mechanism behind this is uncertain.

Chronic Paroxysmal Hemicrania (CPH)

Frequent daily episodes of CPH almost always respond to the use of 25 milligrams of indomethacin (Indocin) taken three times daily (103). This medication, which is more commonly used for joint pains, is best taken after meals, as it may cause indigestion. There are no objections to its use in CPH for prolonged periods of time.

Conclusions

The first step in managing cluster headache is to recognize its specific pattern as distinct from other forms of headache. The medication used to control it is quite different from that prescribed for trigeminal neuralgia and other forms of facial pain, and it is used in a different manner from the medication employed for migraine. Appropriate treatments can help most patients with this very painful and unpleasant disorder. It must be emphasized that all the medications mentioned should only be taken while patients remain under the care of the doctor supervising the entire treatment.

10

NEURALGIA, SINUSITIS, AND A PAIN IN THE NECK

When people say that a headache is caused by "nerves," they usually mean a state of anxiety or nervous tension. Tension headache was the subject of chapter 8. Other types of headache are more literally produced by direct irritation or compression of the nerves supplying the head, face, or neck.

A nerve contains many fibers, most of which are enclosed in an insulating wrapping called a myelin sheath, like wires inside a cable. Each group of fibers comes from a particular area of the body and is responsible for sensation in that area. The nerve fibers that supply sensation to the forehead, cheek, and chin are branches of the trigeminal nerve. They convey sensation from those parts of the face to the central nervous system. Sensation from the back of the head and neck is mediated by activity in the upper cervical nerves which enters the spinal cord, where it is transmitted to other nerve cells and pathways that relay it to the brain.

A nerve conveys its message in responding to any stimulus by setting up an electrical discharge. The electrical discharge, or impulse, passes along the nerve as a signal to the spinal cord or brain stem. The interweaving of nerve pathways in the spinal cord and brain has much in common with electrical and electronic circuits, so that the term "nerve circuits" is often used to describe them.

When a nerve is irritated anywhere along its course, pain may arise at that particular point. More often the pain feels as though it comes from the whole area supplied by that nerve. If, for example, a sinus infection is irritating a nerve deep inside the cheekbone, an ache may be felt not only in the cheek but also in the upper gum and teeth, which are supplied by branches of the same nerve. The site of pain may be further complicated by two different nerves plugging into the same central circuit within the spinal cord or brain. Some of the central fibers concerned with the perception of pain from the forehead loop downward in the brain stem and make connections with the same cells as spinal nerves that enter the cord in the upper part of the neck (Figure 2.1). This may lead to a misinterpretation of the origin of pain. A disk in the upper part of the neck pressing on one of the roots of the spinal nerves can cause pain not only in the neck and back of the head but also in the forehead. This is called referred pain and is caused by the two nerve pathways converging on a single pathway.

The type of pain set up by an abnormality in a nerve or its central connections, called neuralgia, may be jabbing or persistent. Since the trigeminal nerve is responsible for sensations of the face and the front part of the scalp, we can start by considering pain that arises from it.

Trigeminal Neuralgia (Tic Douloureux)

Any pain originating from the trigeminal nerve may properly be called trigeminal neuralgia, and yet the term is usually applied to a particular type of pain, distinctive and devastating, which strikes its victims like lightning. Unlike lightning, it strikes the same place more than once, again and again, until its repeated jabs may drive the patient to despair. Its name is tic douloureux, French for painful spasm, an understated phrase hallowed by several centuries of usage.

Tic douloureux affects women twice as often as men and most commonly starts after the age of forty. The pain is caused by a change in the pattern of impulses in the trigeminal nerve. Instead of the nerve carrying a regular pattern signaling a touch on the face, it fires off a synchronized barrage of impulses that send an inappropriate signal of sudden pain. The pain is often triggered by touching a particular part of the face, or even by wind blowing on the face. It may be brought on by talking, chewing, brushing the teeth, or shaving. The pain most commonly strikes the gum, cheek, or chin as a sudden single stab or repeated stabs (Figure 1.1), although in about 5 percent of cases the forehead may be affected. The important characteristics of the pain are its intensity, its brevity, and its tendency to recur in cycles. There may be spontaneous remissions for months or years before the symptoms return.

What causes this nerve to become hyperexcitable on one side of the face? There is still controversy as to whether it is simply the result of an age change in the nerve cells or whether the nerve fibers are compressed in the majority of cases. Dr. Peter Jannetta, professor of neurosurgery at the University of Pittsburgh, reported his experience of operating on patients twenty-eight to seventy-nine years old with tic douloureux (55). The operation employed a binocular microscope to examine the nerve at the point where it enters the brain stem, an area not seen in conventional operations performed to cut the nerve (Figure 4.3). Of the first one hundred patients, ninety-four were found to have some identifiable source of compression or irritation of the nerve fibers. The most common cause was the progressive lengthening of a branch of an artery as it hardened with age until it touched on the nerve. Dr. Jannetta reported that most of the patients in whom he moved the artery away from the nerve experienced no more pain. This operation involves a major surgical exploration of the brain stem.

There are some patients in whom nerve compression can be suspected clinically because a constant pain persists between the jabs, or part of the face may feel numb or peculiar. In 2 to 3 percent of patients with multiple sclerosis, a condition in which the insulating myelin sheaths around nerve fibers break down in the central nervous system, tic douloureux may occur as a symptom.

In the majority of patients no signs can be found on examination or through special tests to show any structural abnormality. The question then arises about the best way to treat the pain. Before treatment starts, it is worthwhile to have a dental examination, for the pain may be aggravated if the bite is uneven and throws strain on one side of the jaw.

In epilepsy, brain cells fire off synchronously in a manner rather similar to trigeminal nerve cells in tic douloureux. For this reason, antiepileptic drugs are used in the treatment of tic douloureux with considerable success. Carbamazepine (Tegretol) is the medication most often prescribed. It may keep the pain under control indefinitely, but the treatment requires taking pills regularly. Another agent, baclofen (Lioresal), which was introduced for the treatment of spasticity, is also used to lessen the pains of tic douloureux.

If the condition persists in spite of medication, there are two surgical options. One is the Jannetta procedure, an exploration of the brain stem to move away any blood vessels that are pressing on the trigeminal nerve. The vessel is maintained in its new position with a small piece of surgical sponge. Although a major operation, it has the advantage of leaving facial sensation intact. The alternative operation is a simpler and quicker procedure—the insertion of a probe to thermocoagulate the trigeminal ganglion, as described in chapter 9. The aim is to partially destroy the pain fibers while preserving normal touch sensation of the face and, if possible, the protective blink reflex. After this procedure, 2 percent of patients experience troublesome sensations in the partly numb areas. Injecting alcohol or other substances into the trigeminal ganglion or cutting the offending divisions of the trigeminal nerve are other surgical approaches that have been employed in the past.

Glossopharyngeal Neuralgia

This condition is one hundred times less common than trigeminal neuralgia. It affects the nerve that supplies sensation to the back of the tongue and throat, as well as a nearby nerve, the vagus, a branch of which supplies the ear. Its jabbing quality is similar to that experienced in tic douloureux, but the pain stabs the ear and the back of the throat on the same side and is triggered off by talking, swallowing, or coughing. The treatment follows the same principles as that for tic douloureux.

Neuralgia After Shingles (Postherpetic Neuralgia)

The word "shingles" comes from the Latin *cingulum*, meaning a belt or girdle. The condition is the result of an infection of a nerve root, and the resulting blotchy red rash and blisters usually run around half the body like a belt. Shingles may also affect the trigeminal nerve, usually as a strip extending over one side of the forehead (see Figure 10.1). Since the condition may be painful, it comes into consideration as a cause of headache. It is caused by a herpes virus called herpes zoster, hence the name "postherpetic neuralgia." It is the same virus that causes chicken pox. After an attack of chicken pox, the virus persists in the nervous system in a latent state until it is reactivated in later life to cause herpes zoster. Herpes zoster should not be confused with the virus herpes simplex, which causes the common cold sore on the face, or herpes type II virus, which is responsible for genital herpes.

After the rash of shingles subsides, it leaves in its wake a partially numb area that may ache. The virus infection alters the normal composition of fibers in the nerve so that the usual pattern of nerve impulses is out of balance and may be interpreted as pain. The changes caused by the virus extend into the central nervous system, because cutting the affected nerve root does not relieve pain. Corticosteroids such as prednisone are given in the active phase of the illness to ease pain and prevent the neuralgia that may follow the illness (38). This treatment carries a slight risk of spreading the infection, thus producing an attack of chicken pox. It has not had any more serious reactions in people who were otherwise healthy. Once the pain is established it can be treated by local measures, such as the use of vibrators or electrical stimulation over the affected area or repeated intravenous infusions of a dilute solution of a local anesthetic, which often gives some lasting benefit. Some pills that elevate the patient's mood, such as amitriptyline, also have an action on central nerve pathways and diminish the pain. Postherpetic neuralgia is difficult to abolish by any form of treatment; the aim is to lessen the pain's severity to a more tolerable level until it gradually subsides on its own.

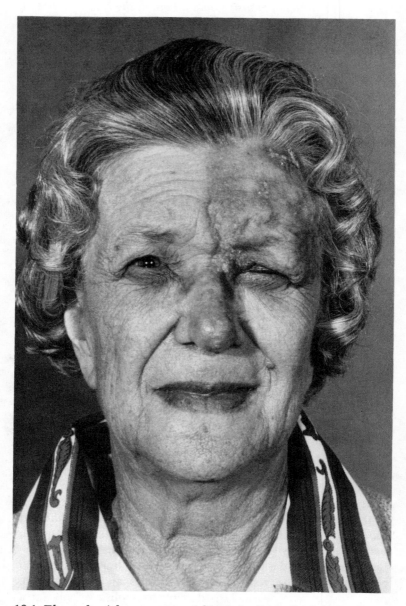

10.1 *The rash of herpes zoster (shingles) affects the left forehead due to infection of the first division of the trigeminal nerve.*

Atypical Facial Pain

The word "neuralgia" is overused and is often applied to any persistent pain in the head or face. Disorders affecting the skull bones may set up neuralgic pains, as may problems with the teeth, sinuses, and other nearby structures. Many of the conditions described as neuralgia in the older medical literature are now known to be variations of migraine and are therefore called facial migraine (or "lower-half headache") or are known to be a form of cluster headache.

One very strange kind of neuralgia has been designated "atypical facial pain" because it is not typical of any of the known causes and its origin is unknown.

The pain is usually felt in the angle of the nose, the upper gum, and the cheek and may arise spontaneously or follow tooth extraction or facial injury. It is constant and penetrating in quality and fluctuates in intensity with the patient's mood. It may be barely noticeable when the individual is occupied and happy and scarcely tolerable when the patient is inactive and disturbed. So closely is the pain bound up with the emotions that it has been regarded as a symptom of a depressive state. This explanation is not entirely satisfactory because the pain persists, at least in some measure, even when the person concerned is relieved of any associated depression. It is a common experience that the condition is not improved by operations on the teeth, nose, or sinuses, or by blocking the various nerves that contribute to the perception of pain from the affected area. Although the face becomes numb, the pain continues. It may be relieved by antidepressant pills, so that the patient can live with the disorder. Electric shock therapy has been reported to cause improvement.

The essential factor for any form of treatment is missing: knowledge of the site of the pain's origin. I suspect that it will be found in the central connections of the second division of the trigeminal nerve, but the condition is rare, and most surgeons are reluctant to perform any operation for a condition that has been considered to exist in the mind rather than in an identifiable part of the brain.

Pain from the Eye

When anyone develops headaches, almost invariably someone suggests the possibility of eyestrain, and a consultation
with an eye doctor follows. What is eyestrain? The term means
that the patient has a refractive error or an imbalance of the
eyes muscles that requires a continual effort to overcome.
Imbalance of the eye muscles means that the eyes tend to drift
inward or outward unless the individual concentrates on keeping the visual axes parallel. We are all familiar with the experience of seeing double when we are tired. The print blurs
and then separates into two images. With a conscious effort we
can bring the images together again. Some people have to make
this effort all the time to keep the eyes aligned. The muscular
activity required for this may set up a headache. The problem
may be helped by eye exercises.

More severe pains can arise from the eye if the pressure
within the eyeball increases (as in glaucoma) or if there is pressure on the eye from a tumor in the eye socket. Some forms of
glaucoma may be mistaken for migraine because pain is felt in
the eye, radiating over the forehead on that side. This can easily
be checked by an ophthalmologist measuring the pressure in
the eyeball.

Sinusitis

There is no mistaking a full-blown attack of acute sinusitis.
The nostril is blocked on one or both sides, and pain extends
over the check or forehead (Figure 1.1). The affected area is
tender when tapped with the finger, and jolting or jarring it
gives rise to pain. The sinuses are air cells present in the bone
of the forehead (frontal sinuses) and in the cheekbone on each
side (maxillary sinus or antrum), while others are situated
deeply behind the bridge of the nose (sphenoid and ethmoid
sinuses). The sinuses are filled with air, and their secretions
drain freely into the nose. They are responsible for the normal
resonance of the voice. If swelling of the mucous membrane
lining the nose occurs, the small openings of the sinuses become
blocked, and their secretions are retained. The voice becomes

dead and lifeless, without its usual timbre, as it does when we have a cold in the nose. If the patient is subject to any changes in air pressure when the sinus opening is blocked, a severe pain may be felt in the forehead or cheek. Anyone who has experienced this when flying will be sure to carry a nasal decongestant spray on future airplane trips.

The treatment of sinusitis requires reestablishing the airway in the nostrils by shrinking the mucous membrane with decongestant drops or spray. It is best to lie on a bed with the head tilted back so that the drops run to the back of the nose where the opening of the sinuses lies. Once the nostril is clear, the patient sits up and bends forward, and then blows the nose gently to try to clear the retained secretions. A good old-fashioned steam inhalation is often helpful, followed by applying dry heat, sitting in front of a radiator or an infrared lamp. Pills containing ephedrine or pseudoephedrine can be taken two or three times during the day to help constrict the blood vessels of the mucous membranes. If the sinuses are severely infected, antibiotics are prescribed as well, but they cannot replace the free drainage of the sinuses into the nostrils. If free drainage cannot be achieved, the sinus may have to be pierced under local anesthetic by an ear, nose, and throat surgeon to form a new opening. In these days of antibiotic therapy, there are still occasional instances of sinusitis or ear infections that have not been treated adequately; such infections can spread to the cranial bones or even the brain. Fortunately, most cases are cured rapidly and completely.

Sinusitis may be present in disguise in a situation that does not suggest any possibility of infection. For example, I have seen a number of patients who have developed over the preceding few days a one-sided headache, radiating backward over the head from the forehead, without any temperature or nasal blockage. Because the headache was made worse by head movement or jolting, both patient and doctor naturally become concerned. Under these circumstances radiology can give the answer, and an X ray may show one or both frontal sinuses filled with fluid. One of my patients complained of a constant pain in the center of the forehead that had been increasing over the past week, again without any nasal symptoms. X rays showed the region normally occupied by the sphenoid sinus, which is tucked away deeply in the center of the skull bones, to be opaque. At first the radiologist was skeptical and thought that the sinus might have been absent from birth in that particular patient, but when the X rays were retaken after the sinusitis had been treated and the headache relieved, they showed that this sinus was indeed present and had cleared completely.

Some patients are said to awaken with a "vacuum headache" if the opening in the sinus is blocked and the air in the sinus is absorbed, leaving a negative pressure inside. This is comparable to the more severe headaches encountered by air travelers experiencing rapid changes in altitude. Various types of pain around the eye and forehead have been ascribed to deviation of the bone plate (nasal septum) that separates the nostrils, or to enlargement of one of the horizontal bones that divide the air stream flowing through the nose into layers. I remain dubious about the nasal origin of most of these pains. I remember attending a meeting where a surgeon stated that he had cured ninety-seven out of one hundred patients of headache by operating on the nose. One of his colleagues whispered to me how extraordinary it was that the only three patients in whom the operation was unsuccessful must have been the ones that he himself had referred to that surgeon, since none of the three had benefited at all from the procedure. The evaluation of surgery or any other measure of treatment for headache must be very carefully compared with the results of other treatments and with the known course of the untreated illness. Headache often improves spontaneously. If the doctor is enthusiastic and the treatment is new, the psychological impact creates a favorable impression. Any benefit may be attributed to the new therapy rather than to the patient's newfound optimism that is really responsible.

Vasomotor rhinitis is the name given to the blockage of one or the other nostril, often alternating, that occurs particularly on lying down when the mucous membrane becomes congested. It is a very common condition and does not appear to give rise to headache unless sinusitis takes over, despite reports to the contrary.

Teeth as a Source of Head Pain

An infected tooth commonly causes localized pain, but pain may be referred to the second or third division of the trigeminal nerve. Thus, an infection of a tooth or a root fragment in the gum may cause pain in the entire lower jaw and lower gum or in the cheek, upper jaw, and upper gum, depending on its location. At the risk of oversimplifying the problem, it can be said that a constant aching pain in the lower jaw is almost always caused by the teeth; in the upper jaw and cheek, sometimes; and in the forehead, never. A routine dental examination may not disclose the trouble, and therefore X rays of the gums and jaws are usually necessary. If the site of pain is in a tooth or is close to the surface of the gum, the pain will often be exacerbated by hot and cold substances in the mouth.

Pain in the ear and temple may be caused indirectly by dental problems, and is often compounded by jaw-clenching in tense or anxious patients. The jawbone is hinged on each side to permit normal chewing movements (see Figure 10.2). If the fingers are placed in front of the ears and slightly below them, one can feel the gliding movement of the jawbone at this point with each bite. When the bite is unbalanced by loss of the molars at the back of the gums, on either one or both sides, the individual has to chew on one side only, or to use the incisor teeth in the front for chewing. Either way, a strain is set up in the jaw joint opposite the side used for chewing. If, in addition, the patient is tense, the habit of clenching the teeth may aggravate that tendency. The joint under constant pressure often becomes painful so that it is tender in front of the ear, and pain radiates up to the temple or down over the face on the affected side. Sometimes the ear may feel blocked and deaf on that side because the tube running from the ear to the nose (the Eustachian tube), which lies behind the jaw joint, becomes obstructed. If the joint deteriorates, a distinct clicking sensation may be felt or heard over it with each biting movement. This constellation of symptoms is known as Costen's syndrome after Dr. James B. Costen of St. Louis, who first described it (23). The treatment is within the province of the dental surgeon, but the problem of

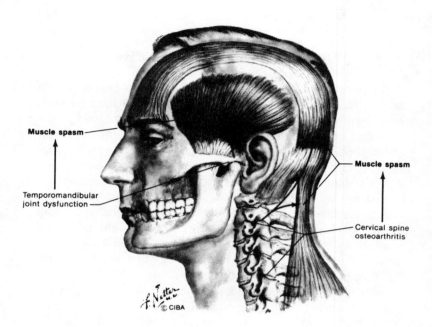

Muscle spasm

Muscle spasm

Temporomandibular
joint dysfunction

Cervical spine
osteoarthritis

10.2 *The hinge joint of the jaw (temporomandibular joint) and the temporal muscle responsible for jaw clenching. Forehead and neck muscles are also shown, along with the fibrous band that joins them together. These muscles can account for a feeling of pressure on top of the head if they are contracted excessively. Reproduced courtesy of Dr. Frank Netter and the CIBA Pharmaceutical Company from* Clinical Symposia, *Volume 33, number 2, 1981.*

nervous tension and jaw-clenching may require additional psychological help and relaxation therapy.

In Costen's syndrome and in jaw-clenchers, the pain may become so severe as to resemble tic douloureux. Some patients with typical tic douloureux are said to respond to a corrected bite, but I have not personally observed this.

Neck Headache

There are a number of ways in which troubles in the neck may cause headache, but, to lay my cards on the table at the outset, I do not consider any of them a very common cause of headache. I have adopted this defensive attitude because there are many who believe that almost all headache comes from the neck and can be cured by its manipulation, just as there are those who believe that most headaches can be cured by nasal surgery, the treatment of allergies, or psychotherapy. Would that it were so simple. If it were, there would be no need for a book of this sort, no need for the classification and diagnosis of headache, and no need for further research into the many different types of headache. Let us look at the ways in which neck disturbances *can* cause headache.

Upper Cervical Syndrome

The neck consists of seven separate bones (vertebrae) separated by disks that act as shock absorbers (see Figures 2.1, 10.3). The bones touch one another at two points where they form joints—first, where vertebral body meets vertebral body

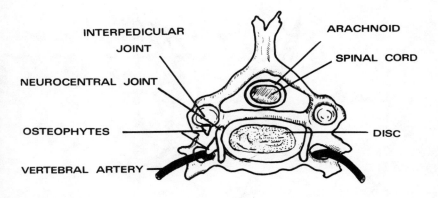

INTERPEDICULAR JOINT

ARACHNOID

SPINAL CORD

NEUROCENTRAL JOINT

OSTEOPHYTES

DISC

VERTEBRAL ARTERY

10.3 *Pressure on nerve roots and the vertebral artery in the neck. A cervical vertebra viewed from above. When a disk between two vertebrae degenerates, bone spurs (osteophytes) project from the interpedicular and neurocentral joints. They may compress the nerve root that runs between them as it leaves the spinal canal on its way from the spinal cord to other structures in the neck. The vertebral arteries are also vulnerable, as they travel in a canal in the bone. The arteries may be narrowed by the pressure of osteophytes when the neck is turned.*

(the neurocentral joints), and second, where the side processes of the vertebrae, which project laterally like wings, connect with one another, resembling the flying buttresses of a cathedral (interpedicular joints). Between the two sets of joints is a gap traversed by the nerves, which pass through to join the spinal cord. Branches of the upper three of these nerves pass over the back of the head (see Figures 2.1, 10.4), while other branches supply the joints of the neck. If the vertebrae are displaced or if the disks degenerate, an arthritic change may take place in one or both types of joint, or the nerve roots may be compressed. When the joints degenerate, they form little spikes of bone termed osteophytes (Figure 10.3). Some osteophytes extend outward from the neurocentral joints, and others extend inward from the interpedicular joints, so that the gap for the

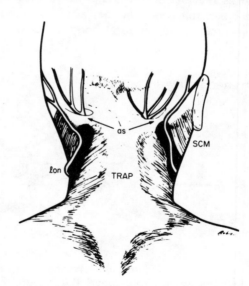

10.4 *The occipital nerves. The greater occipital nerve passes through a gap between the skull and an aponeurotic (fibrous) sling—labeled (as) in figure—before branching over the back of the head. The lesser occipital nerve (lon) is also shown, together with the trapezius (TRAP) and sternocleidomastoid (SCM) muscles. Reproduced from (17), courtesy Dr. Nik Bogduk and ADIS press.*

passage of the nerve root becomes smaller and smaller until the root is compressed. For any of these reasons, nerve impulses may be set up in these roots that give rise to pain over the upper neck and back of the head. Thus the neck has to be considered as a cause of any pain extending over the back of the head, particularly if it is aggravated by neck movement. Some conditions, such as whiplash injury to the neck or rheumatoid arthritis, are particularly liable to affect the upper neck and refer pain to the back of the head.

Neck-Eye Syndrome

A variation on the upper cervical syndrome is a pain shooting to the eye and forehead, related to neck posture. Here, the nerve fibers that have passed through the bone gap to the spinal cord make connection with nerve cells that also receive nerves from the eye and forehead (Figure 2.1). Hence, any sudden movement of the neck can cause a pain in the eye and forehead, even though the origin is in the upper neck. It must be stressed that there is no known way for disturbance of the lower neck to cause pain in the head.

Neck-Tongue Syndrome

In 1980, Dr. Michael Anthony and I described a previously unrecognized syndrome affecting children or young adults on sudden rotation of the neck (66). During strenuous activity such as swimming, tennis, or gymnastics, the patients experienced a sudden pain in the back of the head, associated with a feeling of numbness in that area as well as of the same side of the tongue. This was hard to explain based on conventional knowledge of anatomy. The numbness in the back of the head is easy to understand because bone slippage caused by a sharp movement could stretch part of the second cervical root that carries sensory impulses from that area. But why numbness of the tongue on the same side? To make the story short, it was found that fibers carrying sense of position from the tongue pass from one nerve to another in loops, so that they eventually end up in the second cervical root. Stretching of that C_2 root can thus cause a curious sensation in the tongue. Other reports of this syndrome have appeared since then. Although the syndrome can be caused by disease of the upper cervical spine, the usual occurrence in adolescents seems to result from excessive mobility of the upper neck joint. It is advisable for these youngsters to avoid sports in which there is a risk of neck injury.

Occipital Neuralgia

The greater and lesser occipital nerves supplying sensation to the back of the head (Figure 10.4) feed into the second cervical root. Pain in this area can therefore be caused by disorders of these nerves as well as by strain or compression of the parent root. This sharp and jabbing pain is called occipital neuralgia and is accompanied by tenderness of the nerves on pressure. There may also be numbness or unpleasant sensations in the back of the head on that side (17).

Occipital neuralgia is often caused by a blow to the back of the head or a whiplash injury, but may begin spontaneously. It may respond to treatment with carbamazepine, as does trigeminal neuralgia, and is alleviated temporarily by the injection of local anesthetic, alone or in combination with a long-acting corticosteroid, around the nerve. Immobilizing the neck in a collar, applying localized heat, and physiotherapy may also help. It may become necessary to avulse the offending nerve surgically if pain persists.

"Cervical Migraine"

A form of headache that was thought to be of neck origin and remains controversial is "cervical migraine." The theory behind this concept is based on the fact that the vertebral arteries pass through canals in the neck bones on their way upward to the skull (Figures 6.1, 10.3). If the osteophytes described above extend outward sufficiently from the neurocentral joints, they can push the vertebral artery out of its normal path so that it runs a zigzag course as it ascends. If a person with this problem turns the neck sharply, such as a driver looking backward when backing up the car, the flow in the vertebral arteries may be impaired, a condition called vertebrobasilar insufficiency. This can give rise to a pain in the back of the head together with symptoms coming from the parts of the brain deprived of blood, such as blurred vision or the sensation of flashing lights in front of the eyes, pins and needles around the mouth and down the body, giddiness, slurred speech, loss of balance, and weakness of the legs. The most dramatic example of this I have come across was a man marching past a review point where a dignitary was taking the salute. When the order "eyes right" was given, he turned his head smartly to the right, immediately felt weak in the legs, and fell heavily to the ground.

It has been postulated that the same sort of thing may happen in less dramatic form to patients with moderate degeneration of the neck disks and joints that produces a form of migraine. The theory behind this is that the network of nerve filaments around the vertebral arteries may be stimulated when the artery is compressed by neck movement, thus setting up a slow-motion version of the above symptoms including headache, called "cervical migraine."

There is no doubt that a form of migraine involves the vertebral arteries and the basilar artery that is formed by their junction (described in chapter 4 as "basilar migraine"). What is in dispute is whether degenerative changes in the neck can cause migraine. Basilar migraine occurs most commonly in young women who usually have completely normal necks. Vertebrobasilar insufficiency, on the other hand, usually occurs in older patients who have degenerative changes in the neck but do not suffer from migraine. In our laboratory, we have found that electrically stimulating the nerves that surround the vertebral arteries does not cause much change in the blood flow to the brain.

There have been many claims that migraine can be cured or relieved by manipulating the neck, but a controlled study of mobilization and manipulation of the neck showed that there was no basis for this belief (88). I have certainly seen many patients with migraine and other forms of headache who have not responded to manipulation of the neck. Along with most of my colleagues, I cannot find any real evidence for the concept of "cervical migraine."

Neck Muscle Headache

This is a muscle-contraction or tension headache that occurs when the patient holds the neck stiffly. Many individuals hold their necks rigidly, and this tendency is reinforced if they hear a crackling or crunching noise when they move their necks. This sound is caused by osteophytes at the site of disk degeneration and may induce a feeling of apprehension, so that the neck muscles contract reflexly to stabilize the neck. If patients view their own X rays, without the knowledge that most necks look rather decrepit after a few decades of hard wear, the fear that their neck is degenerating is accentuated, and the neck is held more rigidly than before. Such muscular contraction causes pain in the back of the head as well as in the neck and may spread to involve other scalp muscles, and generalized headache may develop. The management of this problem must include the neck condition as well as the tension state secondary to it.

Conclusions

There are a few headaches that arise from the neck. These may respond to heat, neck traction, neck manipulation, wearing a collar, or injecting local anesthetic or cortisone into the offending joints or nerves. Occasionally they may require an operation to remove disks in the neck or to free or even sever the nerve roots if other measures fail. There are many other forms of headache, the great majority of which bear no other relation to the neck than a certain geographical proximity. These respond to manipulation in direct proportion to the personality of the manipulator and the mystique that surrounds his or her performance.

11

SERIOUS CAUSES
OF HEADACHE

A Box of Bone and Its Remarkable Contents

The skull is a box of bone that opens into the spinal canal through a large opening in its base. The bony framework is lined with membranes containing cerebrospinal fluid; in effect, the brain floats in fluid that helps to support it. The membranes and their contained fluid extend down the spinal canal, cushioning the spinal cord from the bone around it. The crystal-clear fluid is made by the filtering of blood through loops of fine vessels (choroid plexus) contained in two large cavities, one in each hemisphere of the brain, known as the lateral ventricles (see Figure 11.1). The fluid passes from the lateral ventricles into the third ventricle, a slitlike cavity in the center of the brain, and from there flows downward in a canal called the aqueduct (in tribute to ancient Roman plumbing) to the fourth ventricle at the back of the brain. From there the fluid spills out of holes in the sides and back of the fourth ventricle into cisterns surrounding the base of the brain. Some of the fluid then passes into the spinal canal, enclosed by a filmy sheath known as the arachnoid, to bathe the spinal cord. The greater part of the fluid moves up and over the surface of the brain in the subarachnoid space until it reaches a large vein running from front to back at the top of the brain, where the fluid is reabsorbed back into the bloodstream (Figure 11.1). There is thus a continual circulation of fresh fluid through and around the brain. Assuming there is no obstruction to the free flow of fluid, the pressure is determined by the rate of formation and

155

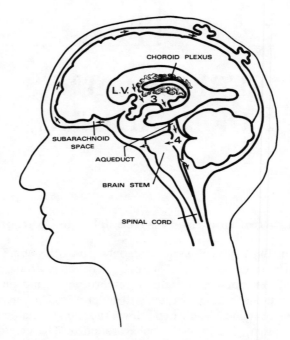

11.1 *The circulation of cerebrospinal fluid. Cerebrospinal fluid is formed by a network of fine blood vessels (choroid plexus) within the cavities (ventricles) of the brain. The fluid passes from the lateral ventricles (L.V.), one on each side of the brain, into the third centricle (3). It flows through the aqueduct into the fourth ventricle (4) and then spills out into the subarachnoid space to bathe the brain and spinal cord. The fluid passes over the surface of the brain (arrows), where it is absorbed into a large vein at the top of the skull.*

reabsorption of the cerebrospinal fluid. If the flow of fluid is interrupted anywhere along its path, the pressure inside the ventricles increases rapidly, a process known as hydrocephalus. In the infant, before the bones of the skull have joined together, the head may grow larger as the result of hydrocephalus. In the older child and adult whose bones have united, the box of bone becomes rigid and cannot expand. The increasing pressure may, however, give rise to headache.

The layers of tissue that wrap around the brain and envelop

it are known as the meninges. There is a hard membrane, the dura, lining the inner surface of the skull. Next comes the arachnoid, named for its likeness to the delicacy of a spider's web, which contains the cerebrospinal fluid. Finally, the pia is attached to the brain and constitutes its containing outer surface. Inflammation of the meninges is known as meningitis and may cause severe headache and stiffness of the neck. Irritation of the meninges by blood spilled into the subarachnoid space from a ruptured blood vessel produces an intense headache of sudden onset that resembles that of meningitis. It may come on so quickly that it feels like a blow on the head. A child with a severe infection of any sort, such as tonsillitis, may develop a headache and stiff neck without any inflammation of the meninges. This is caused by overproduction of cerebrospinal fluid and is called meningism. Sometimes it is difficult to be certain on clinical examination whether a child or adult has meningitis, hemorrhage into the subarachnoid space, or simply meningism. For this reason a CT scan of the brain may have to be performed and a sample of the fluid taken from the spinal canal (by a process known as lumbar puncture) be examined under the microscope and subjected to chemical analysis.

Most remarkable of all the contents of the box of bone is the brain itself. Its convoluted appearance and jellylike consistency may appear to be a frail and undignified vessel to contain the mind of a human being, and yet we live in our brain, and all the other parts of the body are servants to it. The sole purpose of the lungs, heart, and blood vessels is to supply the brain with oxygen and nourishment so that it can think for us. The sole purpose of the bones, joints, and muscles is to provide messengers to do the brain's bidding. The brain contains ten billion nerve cells, interconnected like complex electronic circuitry that would make a computer blanch were it suitably endowed. Regrettably, the brain and modern technology share the attribute of built-in obsolescence. It has been estimated that brain nerve cells die at the rate of about ten thousand each day from the age of sixteen onward. However, a rapid calculation will convince the fainthearted that there are more than enough cells to last a lifetime. Curiously enough, the brain is insensitive to pain, so that diseases affecting it cause headache only when they displace blood vessels or block the flow of fluid, as in the case of brain tumors, or if they irritate the meninges. Encephalitis, or inflammation of the brain, is associated with headache because of swelling of the brain. Since the meninges are often involved as well, viral infection of the brain is usually called meningoencephalitis.

Low-Pressure Headache

If the pressure of the fluid surrounding and supporting the brain is lowered, the brain no longer "floats" at the same level, and strain is then placed on the blood vessels to help maintain its position. This strain results in a headache aggravated by sitting or standing, for the brain tends to sag downward when the head is held upright. Such a headache may develop after a lumbar puncture. Lumbar puncture is a method of sampling the contents of the cerebrospinal fluid by inserting a fine needle between the vertebrae in the lower part of the back (lumbar region). The area is numbed first by the injection of local anesthetic so that the procedure is not as drastic as it may sound. In skilled hands and with a modest degree of luck, the procedure may end with the patient asking, "When are you going to begin?" just as the needle is being removed.

No matter how skilled the doctor, about 10 milliliters of fluid must be withdrawn in order to carry out all the appropriate tests. The patient has to make up that amount of fluid afterward and is advised to rest in bed for twenty-four hours. For the first few hours it is best for the patient to remain in the prone position (lying on the stomach). In this position the small puncture made in the arachnoid is uppermost, and the normal curve of the spine tends to close off the puncture wound. If the patient lies on the back on a soft mattress, the puncture wound may open so that fluid can seep into the tissues. In any event, some patients do develop a headache after lumbar puncture. In this case, the only solution is to lie down and drink plenty of fluid until the cerebrospinal fluid is replenished and the brain floats again in its usual buoyant fashion.

High-Pressure Headache

Any abnormality in the circulation of the cerebrospinal fluid that prevents its flow through the ventricles and canal system of the brain, or a blockage of the great vein that absorbs the fluid, will cause an increase in intracranial pressure. The arteries may be displaced and respond by causing a headache that is exacerbated when bending forward, or when the head is jolted or jarred. This will be discussed in the next chapter, which deals with the question every headache sufferer asks at some time: "Do I have a brain tumor?"

In addition to cerebrospinal fluid outside the brain substance, each cell in the brain contains fluid, and minute quantities of fluid lie between the cells. If the fluid content of the cells increases, the whole brain may swell, increasing the pressure within the skull or cranium. This is known as cerebral edema, or "water on the brain." A 2.5 percent increase in brain water can cause a fourfold increase in intracranial pressure.

Water on the Brain

This expression has fallen from common usage, but the naïve phrase expresses the problem succinctly. I remember a joke from childhood that ran something like this:

> "There I was at the North Pole, face to face with an enormous bear, and had no gun."
> "What did you do?"
> "I hurled an icicle at his head."
> "Did the icicle kill him?"
> "No, but the bear eventually died of water on the brain!"

I wondered then what exactly was meant by water on the brain. I doubt if I would have appreciated the explanation—that the water was not on the brain but in the brain and was indeed contained in each cell of the brain. There are many factors that may help to retain fluid in brain cells. Perhaps we could start with one related to the bear's environment. High doses of vitamin A can cause swelling of the brain. Vitamin A is concentrated in the livers of fish, seals, and animals such as bears and huskies living in the Arctic or Antarctic. You may recall being given cod-liver oil as a child to increase your body stores of vitamins A and D, and adolescents are now given vitamin A as treatment for acne. Sometimes this is used in combination with the antibiotic tetracycline, which can also cause brain swelling—a rare cause of headache, but one to look out for.

Eskimos are well aware of the dangers of eating excessive quantities of liver, but this fact was unknown to some of the early explorers. Four to eight hours after eating a meal of seal liver, the Arctic or Antarctic explorer may experience severe headache, giddiness, vomiting, and diarrhea, followed days later by peeling skin. Sir John Cleland and Dr. R. V. Southcott recount the case of Mawson and his companion, Mertz, who probably suffered from this condition in the Antarctic expedition of 1911–1914 after they were forced to eat their dogs, including the livers. Mertz subsequently suffered vomiting, diarrhea, and delirium. Both were troubled by "wholesale peeling of skin" all over their bodies. Mertz eventually died after a convulsion (22).

Swelling of the brain may be a feature of lead poisoning and has been reported occasionally after treatment with the antibiotic tetracycline, the urinary antiseptic nalidixic acid, and the long-term use of steroids such as cortisone. Brain swelling resulting from steroids is paradoxical, because one of the quickest ways to reduce brain swelling is to give large doses of cortisonelike substances. Either a deficiency or an excess of cortisone, which is made by the adrenal glands, may be associated with brain swelling. Other hormone changes may also be responsible. One of the most interesting is the rare occurrence of brain swelling in plump young women, pregnant women, or women taking the contraceptive pill. There are many other causes of headache, of which this is one of the least common, so there is no need for any woman to leap to the conclusion that she has the most obscure of all the causes. Moreover, when it does occur, it responds so well to treatment that the condition is generally known as benign intracranial hypertension (BIH).

Brain swelling may appear after head injury or brain surgery, or when a large blood vessel to the brain has become
blocked. Prompt control of brain swelling by steroids or by the
intravenous infusion of mannitol or glycerol, which absorb
fluid from the tissues, has been a major factor in improving the
recovery rate in all these serious situations.

Blood Pressure

Our discussion of pressure has so far covered pressure inside
the skull (intracranial pressure), pressure of the fluid surrounding the brain (cerebrospinal fluid pressure), and pressure within
the brain tissue itself. All these are obviously interdependent
and are linked with the pressure in the arteries that supply
the brain with blood, since the arteries provide the only means
for fluid to enter the cranium.

There is no doubt that a sudden increase in blood pressure
to high levels will cause severe headache. In acute nephritis, a
kidney disease, the inflamed kidney manufactures a substance
that causes the blood pressure to rise sharply. Other forms of
high blood pressure may also come on acutely. A small tumor
of the adrenal glands (with the glorious name of pheochromocytoma) can release epinephrine and norepinephrine into the
bloodstream intermittently. When it does, the heart rate increases, possibly felt as "palpitations" in the chest, the hands
become shaky, and the blood pressure shoots up. The patient
commonly feels a sudden sharp ache over the top or in the back
of the head, which does not usually last long, probably because
the blood vessels of the brain and scalp soon constrict in response to the circulating epinephrine, and the patient then looks
pale. This type of headache is remarkably similar to that described in chapter 3 as benign sex headache, occurring at the
moment of orgasm, in which case, too, epinephrine may suddenly be released. A third form of headache in which epinephrine causes an upsurge of blood pressure has been observed
in patients taking MAO inhibitors for depression. The brain's
content of epinephrine, norepinephrine, and serotonin is low
in states of depression. Normally these monoamines are broken

down in the body by monoamine oxidase (MAO), an enzyme. In order to allow the levels of monoamines to build up, this enzyme is put out of action by drugs known as MAO inhibitors. These are extremely effective in improving the patient's mood, but if any substance like epinephrine enters the body or is manufactured in excess inside the body, it cannot be destroyed before it causes an acute rise of blood pressure. Cheese and some kinds of red wine contain chemicals that are either precursors of epinephrine or release it in the body, and these substances are therefore forbidden to any patient taking MAO inhibitors. Before this was recognized, there were reports of patients attending wine and cheese parties who suffered a devastating headache as a result. Any person taking these pills must be extremely careful about taking any other form of medication at the same time. Even inhaling a nasal decongestant may be hazardous, because some nasal sprays contain substances allied to epinephrine. MAO inhibitors are sometimes used for the prevention of migraine and tension headache (discussed in chapters 7 and 8).

Apart from these acute episodes, the relationship between headache and high blood pressure is probably indirect. It is said that people with high blood pressure are likely to awaken in the morning with a headache, but it passes as they get up and move about. Certainly, migraine attacks increase in frequency in patients whose blood pressure rises, and control of the blood pressure subsequently improves the headaches. It is uncertain whether a modest increase in blood pressure will actually induce headaches in an individual who has previously been headache free. Only about one-half of patients with high blood pressure complain of headache, and their pressure readings are no higher than those who are headache free. It is probable that just knowing that one's blood pressure is higher than it should be is sufficient cause to induce a tension headache in some people, and that the caliber of the vessels fluctuates more widely as blood pressure increases, making the individual more susceptible to vascular headaches. Adequate control of blood pressure can therefore be regarded as an important element in the management of headache.

Big Strokes and Little Strokes

A stroke is a "stroke of fate" that leaves someone partially disabled as a result of sudden damage to the nervous system. In practice, the term is usually applied to a blockage of a blood vessel or a hemorrhage into part of the brain, which leaves a patient paralyzed on one side of the body. If the right side of the body becomes weak in a right-handed person, the power of speech may also be impaired, since the connections between the brain and the body are crossed. The left hemisphere of the brain is responsible not only for movement of the right side of the body but also for the planning and execution of the complex intellectual skills of speech, writing, and calculation. The single most common factor leading to a stroke is sustained, untreated high blood pressure, although other factors, such as the level of fatty substances in the blood and hereditary susceptibility, also play an important role.

It is easy to see how a hemorrhage into part of the brain can cause headache, simply by occupying space in one hemisphere that displaces pain-sensitive blood vessels. If blood is spilled into the ventricular system so that it becomes mixed with the cerebrospinal fluid, it will pass down the spinal canal in the subarachnoid space, irritate the meninges, and cause neck pain and stiffness as well as headache. After some days, the blood may gravitate to the lowest part of the spinal canal. It then causes pain in the back and legs by producing a sterile inflammation of the nerve roots. This is called subarachnoid hemorrhage because of the plane into which the bleeding occurs, in which the blood cells mingle with the cerebrospinal fluid. It may complicate any cerebral hemorrhage but is most commonly caused by bleeding from an aneurysm, a "blowout" on an artery.

An aneurysm looks like a small balloon the size of a cherry or even a red currant. Some people are born with these little sacs on the arteries, or at least with a predisposing weakness of the vessel wall, yet they may not cause a moment's trouble. In others, particularly those who develop high blood pressure, the aneurysm may enlarge and eventually rupture, often at a time of strenuous physical exertion. Since the bleeding takes place from a high-pressure system, it is potentially dangerous and requires careful assessment by a neurological unit. A subarachnoid hemorrhage can also arise from a low-pressure system (from abnormal cerebral veins) if the patient happens to be born with a cerebral angioma. An angioma is a collection of blood vessels in which blood passes through large channels from arteries to veins (Figure 12.2). It looks like a cluster of varicose veins on or in the brain. If the doctor listens with a stethoscope over the skull or over the eye, a murmuring sound can sometimes be heard as blood is shunted through large blood vessels in the angioma. The condition may be present throughout life without any complications and, if it does bleed, the hazards are much less than that of an aneurysm because of the low pressure in the system. Much has been written in the medical literature about angiomas underlying migraine-type headache. This does not appear to be a valid relationship, because only 5 percent of patients with proven angiomas have suffered from migraine headache, and this proportion is no greater than that of the general population.

A more common cause of stroke is a thrombosis, or clot, in a vessel narrowed by the accumulation of a fatty deposit called atheroma. Long before any stroke occurs there may be warning symptoms of transient weakness in one side of the body, pins and needles, blurred vision, giddiness, loss of balance, and a host of other temporary disabilities. These symptoms may indicate insufficient blood flow in the cerebral vessels. They are brought into the present discussion simply because they can be accompanied by headache. The ache is in the back of the head, if the vertebral and basilar arteries are momentarily obstructed, or on one side of the head, if flow is suddenly diminished in one carotid artery. The occurrence of odd neurological symptoms in association with headache, particularly a one-sided headache, may suggest the incorrect diagnosis of migraine. The cause of headache in vascular insufficiency is probably dilatation of extra blood channels that open up to bypass the blocked artery and convey blood to the brain through a roundabout route. Vascular insufficiency is treated by opening up the narrowed arteries if the obstruction is in a place accessible to surgery, or, if no surgical measures are possible, by preventing the clumping together of small particles in blood known as platelets, in order to minimize the possibility of a clot forming in the narrowed artery. It appears that an aspirin tablet taken once a day is as effective as any treatment to stop blood platelets sticking together, and this is now being used as part of the treatment.

Many patients with headache fear that they are more liable to have a stroke than their next-door neighbor. This is a groundless fear. Headaches from vascular insufficiency are very uncommon and are associated with other symptoms. Headaches from other causes are legion.

Blood Vessels as a Target

Lack of Oxygen

Much has been said so far about blood vessels. They are pain-sensitive, they may dilate to give rise to headache, and they are very vulnerable to any changes in the blood they carry. Any reduction of oxygen in the bloodstream makes the vessels dilate, which thus increases the blood flow and makes more oxygen available to the tissues. Any accumulation of carbon dioxide has a similar effect but is rather more potent in dilating the vessels. After a convulsion or epileptic fit, in which breathing stops momentarily, the oxygen supply to the brain is reduced for several seconds, and the carbon dioxide level of the blood increases. The vessels therefore dilate and the patient awakens with a headache. In a less dramatic situation, the same mechanism may apply. A crowded meeting in a relatively small room on a winter's night with all the windows closed is a perfect setting for the respiratory seesaw to swing: the oxygen goes down, the carbon dioxide goes up. The vessels dilate and the headache starts. That so many headaches are present on waking in the morning may also be related to the fact that the carbon dioxide content of the blood slowly increases during sleep, causing vessels to dilate. "His face was flushed with sleep." It may soon grow pale with headache.

Any poison that prevents the normal delivery of oxygen to the tissues will have the same effect. Carbon monoxide is the most common example.

In 1931, Charles Kingsford Smith set off to fly from Australia to England in an Avro Avian named Southern Cross Minor in an attempt to break the previous record time for the flight. As he was approaching Rangoon he twice wrote in his logbook that he was suffering from acute headaches and had suffered a spell of dizziness. After leaving Rangoon, he was halfway across the Bay of Bengal when he wrote, "I feel awful! Think I've got a touch of sunstroke." By the time he had reached Calcutta he felt very weak and sick. On arrival at Karachi, he was unable to sleep and recorded that he had "a rotten night . . . my head bashed away like a bloody drum." His illness became worse as the flight progressed until finally he made an emergency landing in Turkey after writing, "I feel as though I might die before this flight is over . . . must find a place to land . . . if I don't I'll crash for sure." After recovering he flew on to Athens, with a recurrence of his symptoms on the way. It was in Athens that the leak in the exhaust pipe was discovered, a leak that had allowed carbon monoxide to diffuse into the cockpit and incapacitate him with headaches and dizzy spells (78).

Low Blood Sugar

Under normal circumstances the brain obtains its energy only from glucose. Severe lowering of blood sugar levels means that the brain cannot obtain nourishment, and the resulting symptoms are similar to those of oxygen shortage. This occurs most commonly in diabetic patients who give themselves more insulin than is necessary for their present diet or take an excessive number of pills to lower the blood sugar. Curiously enough, low blood sugar may follow an excessive intake of sugar or other carbohydrates. This is called carbohydrate intolerance. After a high-carbohydrate meal the blood sugar may rise rapidly but then fall after an hour or two to subnormal levels, causing confusion, trembling, unpleasant abdominal sensations, and headache. The same sequence may be found in patients who have had part of their stomach removed for peptic ulcers.

Vascular headaches, particularly migraine, may be triggered by low blood sugar.

The blood vessels are also a target for any toxins circulating in the body. With most severe infections, a vascular headache contributes to the patient's misery. When there is a reaction to injections of typhoid or smallpox vaccine, a throbbing headache is a common accompaniment. The common hangover headache is a toxic dilatation of intracranial vessels, caused by the breakdown products of alcohol.

Rebound Headache

One interesting cause of headache is the rebound dilatation of vessels that follows the use of any substance causing them to constrict. Any agent that narrows vessels is called a vaso-constrictor, the most common being caffeine. Caffeine is a component of many headache powders or pills. Some people take these as a pick-me-up because of their caffeine content. Caffeine is a stimulant as well as a constrictor of blood vessels. As the effect wears off, the user feels let down. The cerebral vessels then dilate again, a dull headache appears, and the stage is then set for taking a few more pills. This is a vicious cycle of caffeine intake and caffeine-withdrawal headache. The same cycle may trouble habitual coffee and tea drinkers who experience withdrawal symptoms, including headache, if more than a few hours elapse between coffee and tea breaks. Habitual intake of analgesic tablets, whether or not they contain caffeine, is potentially dangerous because their use over a number of years can cause permanent damage to the kidneys.

Drugs

Some medications are given deliberately to cause dilatation of arteries and so may evoke headache as a side effect. Amyl nitrite or nitroglycerin (glyceryl trinitrate) is given to patients whose coronary arteries are narrowed sufficiently to cause pain or tightness in the chest upon exertion (angina pectoris). The pills are effective in easing the chest discomfort but may cause a throbbing headache. Workers who come into contact with nitroglycerin, other nitrates, or other vasodilator substances may complain of headache. Histamine dilates vessels and has been used experimentally to induce headaches in order to study the effects. It is possible that histamine release in allergic reactions may sometimes account for headache. Certain drugs cause headache as a side effect, particularly those that dilate vessels, such as dipyridamole. Of patients who are being treated regularly with indomethacin, an agent most effective for the relief of arthritis and other joint and muscle pains, and indeed for some types of headaches, 25 percent notice a continual dull headache.

Meningitis and Encephalitis

Arteries dilate as a part of the inflammatory process, such as an infection of any part of the body. The blood supply to the affected area is thus increased, allowing the white cells of the blood to flock to the area to aid in the body's defenses. Those white cells that die while struggling with the invaders accumulate as pus. Any inflamed area becomes tense because the dilated vessels leak fluid into the tissues at the site of battle between the infecting organism and body cells. The vessels are thus dilated and displaced by tissue swelling so that they are very sensitive to pressure or to jolting and jarring.

Meningitis is an inflammation of the membranes of the brain, usually caused by bacteria, and starts as a severe headache with neck stiffness, fever, and usually aversion to light (photophobia). The diagnosis may be confirmed through a sample of the cerebrospinal fluid by lumbar puncture, and the appropriate antibiotic is then prescribed. The infection gains access to the nervous system through the bloodstream but may also invade directly from the ear, nose, or sinuses. In the fifth century B.C., Hippocrates warned that an association of fever with acute pain in the ear was to be dreaded, "for there is danger that the man may become delirious and die" (3).

Encephalitis is an infection of the brain itself. It may be an extension of meningitis or may be a viral infection that attacks the brain cells directly. The symptoms are much the same as meningitis, but earlier in the disease the patient becomes mentally confused and drowsy.

There is a much milder and more common form of viral infection called either viral meningoencephalitis because the membranes of the brain and the brain tissue are both involved, or aseptic meningitis because no bacteria can be grown from the fluid. Most severe viral infections cause some degree of meningoencephalitis. Most children and adults experience headaches with measles, mumps, and influenza, and when the cerebrospinal fluid has been examined at this time, an increase in the number of cells in the fluid indicates that the virus is active in the nervous system. Most of these viral illnesses subside without any complications, and many require no treatment other than bed rest and analgesics to relieve headache. The number of serious cases of encephalitis is fortunately small. The persistence of any headache with a fever is nevertheless a reason to call the doctor to see whether further diagnostic tests or active treatment are necessary.

Headache at Retiring Age

A particular form of headache that usually affects patients over the age of fifty-five is caused by an inflammation of blood vessels in the scalp and often in the cerebral vessels as well. The condition is known as temporal arteritis or giant-cell arteritis. It is worth special mention because it is so uncommon that it may not be thought of until the condition is well advanced, and early treatment is essential in preventing complications that may be serious enough to progress to blindness.

Temporal arteritis is a low-grade inflammation of arteries that usually affects the scalp vessels first, particularly the arteries in the temple, hence its name. The walls of the arteries become thickened and packed with inflammatory cells including giant cells containing many nuclei, which gives rise to the alternative name, giant-cell arteritis. It may be accompanied by redness, swelling, and tenderness of the arteries in the scalp (see Figure 11.2), in which case there is little difficulty in diagnosis. The more difficult diagnostic problems are those where the symp-

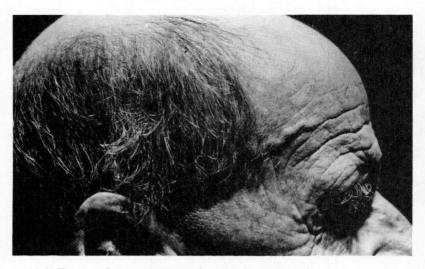

11.2 *Temporal arteritis. Branches of the temporal artery may be swollen, tender, and pulseless, as this photograph displays, but the condition is not always so obvious. On the other hand, many people have naturally prominent temporal arteries.*

toms are simply a dull, persistent ache on one or both sides of the head. To complicate the issue, arteries in other parts of the body may be involved, in which case the first symptoms may be a general rundown feeling, together with aches and pains in the muscles and joints, like a low-grade influenza. This condition has been called polymyalgia rheumatica, meaning rheumatic aches in the joints and muscles. One rather distinctive symptom of temporal arteritis is aching of the jaw muscles when chewing. This is caused by reduction of the blood supply to these muscles as the arteries become narrowed.

The development of these symptoms or of headache in this age group warrants a blood count and estimation of the sedimentation rate of the blood. Blood cells sediment or separate out under the influence of gravity if blood is left standing in a test tube with a substance to prevent it from clotting. This separation can be seen quite easily as a band of clear plasma above the dense red color of the packed cells. Normally the cells sediment at less than 20 millimeters each hour, but in inflammatory conditions like temporal arteritis the rate is usually more than 40 millimeters each hour, and may be as fast as 100 millimeters in one hour. This simple test can help confirm the suspicion of temporal arteritis. To make completely certain of the diagnosis, it is usually necessary to remove a small section of an affected scalp artery and examine it under a microscope.

It is most important to diagnose the condition early, because it may spread to intracranial arteries. Unfortunately, it has a predilection for picking out the ophthalmic artery, which supplies the retina of the eye. If this artery is affected, it may clot in that eye, and vision may be lost. This can happen with appalling suddenness. A wise old dairy farmer was sent to me after having lost his eyesight in the right eye only a few days after developing a headache in the right temple. He had virtually made his own diagnosis. He said to me, "You know, it's a funny thing, but the pulse in my right temple just disappeared at the same time as I went blind in the right eye." This tragedy can often be avoided by starting treatment with steroids as soon as the diagnosis is made. It may be necessary to continue treatment for twelve months or more to hold the condition at bay while it burns itself out.

Conclusions

We have dealt with a large number of problems, some minor and some major, that can affect the magic contents of the white box of bone to produce headaches. Others will be considered in the next chapter on brain tumors and other lumps or bumps which may occupy space in that unyielding box where space is at a premium. Fortunately, nasty causes of headache are rare, but we must never relax our vigilance so that we can spot them before they have time to do any harm.

12

DO I HAVE
A BRAIN TUMOR?

How Common Is Brain Tumor
as a Cause of Headache?

Not all patients with brain tumors complain of headaches, and certainly only a very small proportion of those with headaches turn out to have tumors. When a headache clinic was established in our hospital in the 1960s, we made a careful survey of the diagnoses in the first one thousand patients who had suffered from chronic headaches—that is, a headache problem of long duration. Of these, only one was found to have a cerebral tumor. The figures clearly show that patients who have suffered from headaches for five, ten, or fifteen years are extremely unlikely to have a brain tumor and that, if they do, it may well be a coincidental finding not related to the complaint of headache.

Brain tumors are really quite uncommon. They constitute about one-fifth of all tumors in childhood, but in this age group tumors of any kind are fortunately rare. In adults, only 1 percent of all tumors are found in the brain. What are the chances of an individual developing a brain tumor? To take the highest possible incidence first, about 2 percent of all routine postmortem examinations show a brain tumor to have been present during life. Many of these are small and have not given rise to any symptoms during life. Others are secondary deposits that have arisen from some other part of the body and have not grown primarily in the brain. In a sample population, the chance of anyone having any sort of tumor affecting the brain or spinal cord is about one in two thousand (19).

172

The important task for the doctor is to identify the pattern of headache and the associated symptoms that give rise to the suspicion of a tumor. Patients with these symptoms may be given special tests, which will be described later. Those who have a pattern of headache completely different from that of brain tumors may not require any investigation at all. Whether the possibility of tumor is excluded on clinical grounds or by the results of special tests, it is important that patients be completely reassured that there is no serious cause for their headaches.

Types of Brain Tumor

Tumors may be benign or malignant, primary or secondary, operable or inoperable. A tumor is a collection of body cells that multiply indiscriminately without the control or organization that characterizes normal growth. A tumor is said to be benign if it grows slowly, pushing other tissues aside, and confines its development to a single site. If the tumor grows rapidly and invades and destroys normal tissues, it is said to be malignant. Fragments of malignant tumors may separate and travel elsewhere in the body by way of the lymph ducts or the bloodstream to set up colonies of abnormal cells, known as secondary tumors. The malignant process in general is called cancer.

Many benign tumors of the brain can be completely removed with excellent results by a neurosurgeon. Examples of these are tumors arising from the meninges, called meningiomas (accounting for some 20 percent of all brain tumors), tumors of the pituitary gland (about 8 percent of the total), cysts above the pituitary gland (3 percent), and fibrous growths on the eighth cranial nerve, the nerve of hearing (8 percent). Some tumors that have all the characteristics of a benign tumor nevertheless lie deeply within the brain or infiltrate between normal structures so that their complete removal would result in severe damage to the brain. They may therefore be inoperable, although classified as benign. Most of these tumors grow from the glial (connective tissue) cells of the brain, which perform a supporting function for the nerve cells, and are therefore called gliomas. Glial-cell tumors range (in microscopic appearance) from benign to highly malignant. They account for about 45 percent of all brain tumors. About 8 percent of brain tumors turn out to be secondary deposits from cancer elsewhere in the body, particularly from the lung (which is responsible for 65 percent), breast, gastrointestinal tract, and kidney.

The task of the neurologist and neurosurgeon is first to determine whether or not a brain tumor is present. If a tumor is then found, they must localize it carefully and determine its nature to ascertain whether or not it can be completely or partially removed without avoidable damage to normal tissues. It is desirable to make the diagnosis as soon as possible, although in most cases it is true that a tumor which can be successfully removed today could be as successfully removed in a few months' time. This may not hold true if the growth of the tumor has imperiled vital structures, which can make operating a matter of urgency. Some tumors in particular must be diagnosed early to obtain the best results. One such example is an eighth-nerve tumor, which causes loss of hearing in one ear years before it produces headache. It should be diagnosed when investigating the deafness and not left to wait for headache or other symptoms to arise. Some brain tumors do have headaches as a main symptom.

A Sinister Pattern of Headache

A brain tumor does not cause headache until it pushes arteries aside, thus placing them under tension, or until it increases intracranial pressure by other means. In some parts of the brain a tumor may grow to a considerable size without doing either of these things. If, on the other hand, the tumor lies in or around the ventricles or aqueduct through which the cerebrospinal fluid flows (Figure 11.1), it causes distension of the ventricles. The blood vessels around the ventricles are displaced, and headache appears as an early symptom. Headache is a feature sooner or later in 90 percent of brain tumors. The pain may be felt in the front or back of the head or in the whole head. It is usually intermittent and does not often approach the intensity of severe migraine, meningitis, or subarachnoid hemorrhage, described in the previous chapter. The ache is commonly made worse by coughing, sneezing, or straining, but this may also be a feature of any intracranial vascular head- ache, including hangover headache. The most distinctive fea- ture of this headache pattern is that it arises in a person not previously subject to headaches or one who experiences a complete change in the pattern of any preexisting headache. The headache also progressively becomes worse (Figure 1.2). If, in addition, the patient yawns or becomes drowsy at in- appropriate times, or develops any symptoms of neurological damage, the suspicion of a tumor greatly increases.

Almost always, some form of neurological deficit accom- panies the growth of a brain tumor. Some deficits may be obvious, such as a progressive weakness or numbness of one side of the body, impaired vision, speaking difficulty, or loss of balance. More subtle may be loss of the olfactory sense, the gradual onset of deafness in one ear, impairment of mental faculties, or bursts of irrational behavior. One patient of mine, a young man whose demeanor had previously been impeccable, was visiting Singapore when he startled his friends, as well as the hotel management, by dropping "water bombs" from his hotel room onto guests relaxing on the lawn below. He followed this by throwing empty bottles down an elevator shaft. Such episodes led to his premature return to Sydney, where a tumor of the frontal brain lobes was diagnosed. Any sudden, drastic alteration of behavior should lead to suspicion of a brain tumor, although there are, of course, many other possible explanations. The association between any of the above symptoms and head- ache is not in itself significant, because other disorders such as migraine can be responsible for many perturbing alterations of brain function preceding or accompanying headache. The sig- nificant aspect of the brain tumor story is the steady worsening of the headache and neurological impairment. Epileptic fits accompanied by headache is a combination that also warrants a thorough investigation.

Some Special Investigations

Must I Be a Guinea Pig?

After the most painstaking examination, it is still not possible to be dogmatic about the presence or absence of a brain tumor. If there is an obvious abnormality found on examination, the likelihood may be very high. Swelling of the optic nerve head (papilledema) may be seen on looking at the interior of the eye with an ophthalmoscope. This indicates that the ophthalmic veins are not able to drain the fluid away from the retina, a sign of increased intracranial pressure. In itself it does not give any clue as to why the pressure is increased. Other signs may enable a neurologist to point precisely to the site of the disturbance, but not to be certain what it is. Special investigations have to be made in order to confirm the location of the abnormality, to assess its size, to see how it is affecting neighboring structures, and to take steps toward determining its nature. After all, even detectives have to take fingerprints.

Patients' reactions to undergoing further tests vary; some are eager to resolve any questions, but others are defensive about their role in the testing process. Variations on the theme of "Must I be a guinea pig?" are common. There is no question of any person undergoing these tests as a guinea pig. Any neurological or neurosurgical team of even modest size conducts these tests regularly with a precision that makes them little more adventurous than taking a ride in a train, and in most cases less hazardous than driving one's car to the hospital. The first series of tests described can be done on an outpatient basis and carries no risk whatever. Specialized X rays of the arteries to the brain are virtually free of risk to anyone who does not have preexisting disease. If there is disease of the arteries or brain, any risk is minimized by conducting the tests in a logical and orderly sequence. Such a risk is small indeed, compared with the benefit of knowing precisely where the trouble lies and what must be done about it.

The Electroencephalogram (EEG)

The EEG or brain-wave test is a fairly simple and routine procedure that is used in the diagnosis of headache if there is an associated problem such as epilepsy. Electrodes are placed on the head with a little paste to ensure that they make good contact with the scalp. Activity of brain cells is associated with electrical changes. When groups of cells become synchronized in their activity, the electrical waves are large enough to be recorded from the scalp. The resulting brain waves are amplified and then recorded automatically by pens on a moving chart. There is no way that electricity can jump back from the machine to shock the patient.

Normally, a rhythm of electrical waves of about ten waves a second, called alpha rhythm, is recorded symmetrically from the back half of the head overlying the part of the brain concerned with sight (the visual cortex). If the eyes are closed, the cells all beat together, like an engine idling in neutral, and the alpha rhythm is picked up. When the eyes are open, each cell has its own task to do, and so the group activity is less conspicuous. The patient is therefore asked to open and close the eyes at intervals throughout the recording, and the alpha rhythm waxes and wanes as a result. An abnormality may show up in the record as an asymmetry in the alpha rhythm, or as slower rhythms classified as theta and delta. These may be localized to a particular electrode, indicating a disturbance in that region of the brain.

After the routine recording is completed, the patient is asked to breathe rapidly and deeply for two or three minutes. This washes carbon dioxide out of the lungs and lowers the level circulating in the blood throughout the brain. The blood level of carbon dioxide regulates the caliber of cerebral blood vessels. If the level goes up, the circumference of the arteries increases so that more blood can flow through them. This is called a vasodilator effect. If the level drops, the circumference decreases so that less blood can pass through (vasoconstrictor effect). Overbreathing lowers the carbon dioxide content in the blood, which in turn reduces the blood flow through the brain.

This is why we may feel faint and dizzy after breathing too much. Any abnormality in the brain waves becomes more obvious when the blood flow slows down.

Near the end of the EEG recording, light may be flashed in the eyes to alter the brain rhythm. The effect of this strobo-scopic light is not unpleasant to most people, who are usually intrigued by the colored patterns they see while the light flashes. The reason for this is that the cells of the visual cortex respond together to each flash of light and beat in unison. The faster the light flashes, the faster the brain cells respond, causing us to "see" a changing spectrum of colors.

Before the days of isotope scanning and computerized X-ray scanning, which will be described shortly, the EEG was the most useful screening test for a brain tumor. It still gives considerable information, particularly if the patient has had any form of epileptic fit, and is complementary to the other tests. The procedure takes thirty to sixty minutes to complete. The recording time varies in each laboratory.

Plain X Rays

The chest is usually X-rayed because a primary cancer of the lung can be responsible for secondary tumors in the brain, and other diseases, like tuberculosis, may also affect both sites. The information obtained from an X ray of the skull is limited. Routine X rays simply show the bones. Any part of the brain that contains calcium also stands out clearly in the X ray. Most tumors do not alter the appearance of bone and therefore do not show up in a plain X ray. The pineal gland, a vestigial structure in the center of the brain, often becomes calcified. It then becomes clearly visible on the skull X ray and indicates whether the midline of the brain is still lying in its normal position or whether it has been pushed out of place by a tumor. Some tumors may absorb calcium, particularly if they are growing slowly. In this case, their position can be seen clearly in plain films of the skull, and some deductions can be made about the type of tumor from the pattern of the calcification. With the advent of computerized axial tomography scanning, the need for plain X rays of the skull has diminished.

Computerized Axial Tomography (CAT or CT Scanning)

The coming of age of the computer provided a means of obtaining much more information from an X-ray beam than was formerly possible. A conventional X ray cannot give a three-dimensional picture because both sides of the skull and all the structures between them are traversed by the X-ray beam. A more precise method of radiography, known as tomography, enables an X-ray beam to focus on a particular plane of the skull, but it cannot display changes in the brain substance.

The EMI Research Laboratories in England devised a way of overcoming this problem in a way that has revolutionized neurological diagnosis. The invention, computerized axial tomography, relies on a narrow beam of X rays that traverses the skull in a series of steps. Two accurately aligned detector units follow the X-ray beam across the head, sensing the transmitted X rays. A reading for each position is recorded, calculated by the computer, and printed out or displayed as a picture. In this way small percentage variations of the X-ray penetration can be perceived, which enables the shadows of the ventricles to be seen and the densities of the gray and white matter of the brain to be distinguished (see Figure 12.1). By this method the position and size of a brain tumor can be discovered without risk to the patient, with little more time spent than with conventional methods, using a comparable amount of radiation. A contrast medium is usually injected into a vein to show abnormalities of the blood vessels or blood-brain barrier. The only possible risk of the procedure is an allergy to their contrast medium. Although the equipment is expensive, the test saves money in many instances by reducing the need for other tests, some of which require hospitalization.

Magnetic Resonance Imaging (MRI) Scanning

This technique is used to obtain an image of the brain or other parts of the body and is derived by applying an external magnetic field that orients hydrogen ions (contained in water) in the direction of the field. It is particularly useful for showing the white matter of the brain and gives better pictures of certain

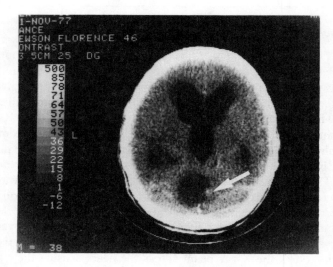

12.1 *Computerized axial tomogram (CAT scan) of the brain. In this case, the ventricles are enlarged because the aqueduct is blocked by a large cystic tumor. The active part of the tumor is seen as a small white dot in the wall of the cyst (arrowed). A surgical procedure easily removed it.*

areas, such as the brain stem, than CT scanning. It is used more for the diagnosis of neurological disorders, such as multiple sclerosis, than in the investigation of headache.

Isotope Scanning (Radionuclide Brain Studies)

This technique, which relies on the injection of a radioactive substance into an arm vein and the uptake of this substance by a cerebral tumor, is now used only occasionally, because CT scanning provides much more information.

Arteriography (Angiography)

In order to see the precise position of the arteries that supply the brain and to pick up any abnormality in them or in the areas they supply, it is necessary to inject a substance into the bloodstream that provides enough contrast on the X rays so that the arteries and veins will stand out clearly against the background of the surrounding skull bones. This procedure is called arteriography or angiography. It is used to detect narrowing of blood vessels (by fat deposits, atheroma), local dilatations on blood vessels (aneurysms), or a congenital abnormality of blood vessels (angioma) (see Figure 12.2). It also points up any displacement of blood vessels from their normal position and may show a network of fine blood vessels within a tumor. The injected dye may linger within an abnormal area to show up as a "blush" after the remainder of the dye has passed through into the draining veins, thus highlighting the tumor.

This method requires hospitalization because the dye is injected into an artery, usually through a thin plastic tube (catheter) inserted into a groin artery. The procedure may be

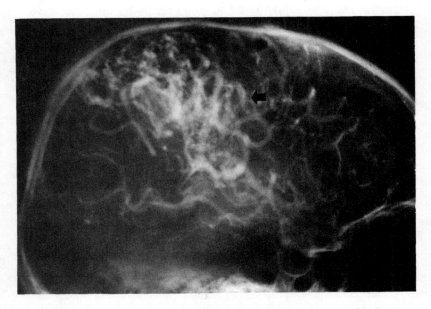

12.2 *Cerebral angiogram. The arteries to the brain are highlighted by means of a dye injected into the arterial system. An arteriovenous malformation (angioma) is indicated by the arrow.*

done under a local or, occasionally, general anesthetic. The patient is usually kept in bed for the following twenty-four hours to ensure that there is no complication at the site of injection. The dye contains iodine and therefore has to be used with caution in anyone allergic to it. Arteriography carries little risk for patients with healthy arteries, but in older patients with degeneration of the blood vessels it may precipitate clotting of a cerebral artery or of the artery into which the injection is made. The complication rate may arise to about 3 percent in this group of patients with known vascular disease.

Arteriography (angiography) has also entered the computer age. By a technique known as digital subtraction angiography (DSA), much smaller doses of dye can be used if injected into the artery, and quite reasonable pictures can be obtained if the dye is injected into a vein. The computerized equipment enhances the image of the small amount of dye circulating to the brain. The end result is not as good as if the injection were made directly into the artery, but its advantage is that a hospital stay is not required. Examples are shown in Figures 12.3a and 12.3b.

Air Encephalography

The fluid-containing channels within the brain—the ventricles, aqueduct, and cisterns—stand out clearly in X rays when outlined by air. For this purpose air can be inserted into the fluid to gain information about the size, position, and shape of the ventricles or to see whether there is any obstruction to the free flow of fluid. This technique is required only rarely, since CT scanning also shows the ventricles clearly.

If intracranial pressure is increased because of a tumor or other abnormality, a neurosurgeon can make a small hole in the skull and place a fine needle into one ventricle with the patient under anesthesia. This serves a dual purpose by reducing the intracranial pressure and injecting air directly into the ventricles in a safe manner. The process is known as ventriculography. A liquid that shows up on X rays can also be injected if the site of obstruction to the fluid-conducting pathways is still in doubt. This substance diffuses through the fluid and outlines the area of obstruction.

What If I Do Have a Brain Tumor?

This section will apply to very few individuals. Most patterns of headache are clearly recognizable as migraine or tension states. If your headache problems have come on recently, are becoming more frequent and severe, and are aggravated by coughing or sudden head movement, then you should certainly consult your doctor, who will refer you to a neurologist if necessary. After a careful examination, it is quite possible that a CT scan will be suggested. Should the results be normal, the cause of your headache is unlikely to be a tumor, since 90 percent or more tumors are picked up by the CT scan.

If a tumor is found, you must then be guided by the neurologist or neurosurgeon who is looking after you. Many types of tumors are benign and may be removed completely with no complications afterward. These include meningiomas, pituitary tumors, and some cystic tumors. An eighth-nerve tumor also may be removed easily with very little risk if diagnosed early, but the dangers of the operation increase with the size of the tumor. If the tumor is large enough to compress the vital parts of the brain that maintain respiration, heart rate, and blood pressure, operation becomes hazardous. Some gliomas, such as the cystic gliomas found in the cerebellum in the rear compartment of the skull, may be cured completely by operating. These are a particularly common form of brain tumor in children. Other gliomas may advance rapidly and be inoperable. In between these extremes there are many that can be partly removed. Radiotherapy or chemotherapy may be used afterward to retard the growth or destroy remaining tumor cells. Such therapy minimizes or delays a possible recurrence.

About 8 percent of brain tumors are secondary deposits from cancer located elsewhere in the body. If there is a single secondary deposit in a position in the brain accessible to the neuro-

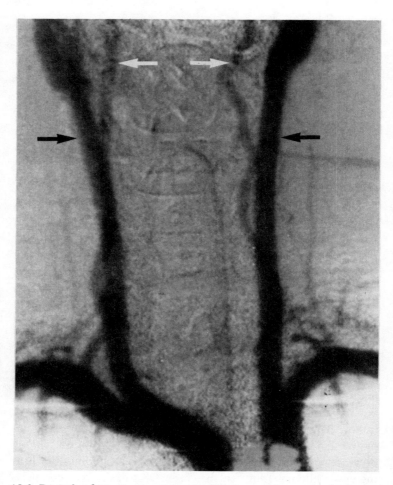

12.3 *Digital subtraction angiogram. All the arteries to the brain are shown together by means of a dye injected into the venous system, with the contrast enhanced by computer. (a.) View of the neck, with the carotid arteries indicated by black arrows and the smaller vertebral arteries by white arrows.*

surgeon, it may warrant removal, although the odds are that there will be other secondary deposits elsewhere in the body. We all know of some patients who have not had any recurrence after an operation on a secondary tumor. There is an unexplained immune process that sometimes steps in to produce a "miracle cure" in some patients with cancer. Unfortunately, this does not happen very often but is frequent enough to give research workers hope that this process might eventually be simulated by treatment in all cases.

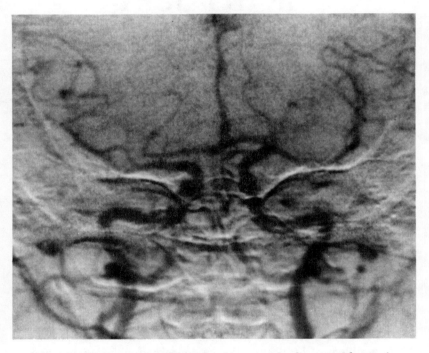

(b.) The skull, viewed from the front, with the carotid arteries branching into the anterior cerebral arteries that run upward in the midline and the middle cerebral arteries that splay outward on each side.

13

HEADACHE AFTER HEAD INJURY

The Nature of the Problem

The faster and farther people travel, the more likely they are to injure their heads. Increasing industrialization adds its share of blows on the head, mitigated to some extent by the use of safety helmets. Head injury may result in a temporary loss of consciousness (concussion), compression of the brain by an enlarging blood clot, or destruction of part of the brain by direct violence. A fracture of the skull itself may not cause any damage to the brain. However, if bone fragments are forced inward, they may press on the brain surface; or, if the line of fracture runs across a large blood vessel in the skull bones and tears it, the brain may be compressed by hemorrhage. Head injury may also disturb the regulation of cerebral and scalp vessels in a way that is still not fully understood.

There are many aspects of head injury that do not relate to the problem of headache. We are concerned with patients who have experienced a head injury that may or may not have knocked them unconscious, who then recover completely without any obvious damage to the nervous system, and yet who complain of frequent headaches, which they attribute to the injury. What part is played by a change in sensitivity of nerves and vessels from damage incurred at the time of the accident? What part is due to the state of anxiety and depression that often follows an accident, particularly one involving the head? Finally, what part can be blamed on the protracted litigation, which so often follows an accident, in attempting to assess whether the symptoms are the result of the accident and whether an insurance company or someone else has a financial liability?

The Size of the Problem

The incidence of post-traumatic headaches varies from 33 to 80 percent in various samplings. A 1944 study from Boston found that a headache lasting more than two months was uncommon in those patients who were dazed but not disoriented after the injury and in those who had little or no loss of memory for the period immediately following the injury (post-traumatic amnesia). The incidence of headache was higher in those patients whose scalp was lacerated. It was also higher in those who had a basically nervous disposition, those with symptoms of anxiety after the accident, and those with occupational difficulties or with pending litigation. Neither the length of time the patient was unconscious nor the existence of a skull fracture seemed to have any correlation with headache (18).

Concussion

An individual who loses consciousness for a minute or two after a blow on the head and then recovers is said to have been concussed. The mechanism is still not completely understood, but it is clearly related to the movement of the brain within the skull. If the skull is crushed by some action while the head remains in a fixed position—for example, by a car sliding off a hydraulic jack, so that part of it rests on the head of the mechanic—the skull may be fractured while the patient remains conscious. A small missile may penetrate the skull without consciousness being impaired. On the other hand, if the skull of a person moving at thirty miles an hour or more hits a telephone pole, the skull decelerates instantaneously to zero. The brain continues to move in relation to the skull until it, too, decelerates to zero. Apart from causing direct damage to the surface of the brain, the sliding movement of the brain exerts a shearing strain on the brain stem, which is relatively fixed in position.

The center for maintaining the brain in a state of awareness is situated in the upper part of the brain stem, in the line of maximum stress. The strain of the impact thus gives a knockout blow to this vital center, so that consciousness is lost.

Some minutes after regaining consciousness it is quite common for the individual to complain of a throbbing head- ache, which is exacerbated when the head is jarred or moved. The majority of people admitted to a hospital with concussion do not complain of headache in the immediate period after injury. A study conducted at the Radcliffe Infirmary, Oxford, England, found that some 60 percent of patients did not ex- perience headache at all while in the hospital, and only 11 percent complained spontaneously of headache or required analgesics for it (110). Then why is it that headaches arise some days or weeks after the injury?

The early treatment of concussion may be important in reducing the disability that so often follows. A group of neuro- surgeons from Helsinki contrasted the results of an active treat- ment program with the routine treatment of comparable patients in the same hospital (94). Members of the active treatment group were visited daily, and the nature of the injury was ex- plained to them. They were encouraged to get out of bed and start physiotherapy. When they attended the follow-up clinic, they were seen by the same doctor who had looked after them in the hospital. The active treatment group returned to work in an average of eighteen days, compared with thirty-two for the others.

It has been found that recovery from a football or other sporting injury is much more rapid and complete than after a traffic accident or an injury at work. The desire for monetary compensation is not the only factor involved in this. The force involved in the latter forms of head injury is usually much greater than blows acquired on the sporting field.

Progressive Headache After Injury

Every now and then one reads a story in a newspaper de- scribing a schoolboy who was knocked unconscious for a few minutes while playing football, was sent to bed at home or boarding school apparently recovered, and was found dead in bed the next morning. The reason for such a tragedy is that the meningeal arteries that lie in the skull may bleed if a fracture line runs across them. Even without a fracture, veins that bridge the gap between the surface of the brain and the inner wall of the skull may be torn and bleed while the subject is completely unaware of it. The onset of headache within minutes or hours of a head injury should cause concern if it progressively worsens or if the patient also becomes drowsy. A hemorrhage of this kind may develop between the skull bone and the dura that lines it (extradural hematoma) or under the dural membrane (subdural hematoma). In either situation the hemorrhage expands, compresses the brain, displaces vessels, and causes headache. The condition requires immediate neurosurgical attention so that the clot can be removed and the pressure relieved.

A slow-motion subdural hemorrhage may cause trouble weeks or months after a head blow, which may have been so mild as to have been forgotten by the time the headache starts. The headache progressively worsens and may be associated with drowsiness in a manner similar to that described for cerebral tumor. The important thing is to be aware of the possibility. Surgical treatment is easy once the diagnosis is made.

Vascular Headaches

Once we have excluded cerebral compression from an expanding clot, we are left with a variety of headaches. These are aften grouped together with giddiness and anxiety symptoms in the postconcussional or post-traumatic syndrome. Dr. Harold G. Wolff considered that there were three main causes of headache in this syndrome. The first was a form of chronic muscle contraction or tension headache, the second was a local ache caused by scar tissue at the site of injury, and the third was a vascular headache resembling migraine. The latter was often one-sided and associated with nausea, vomiting, and distension of the scalp arteries in the manner of migraine. It is probable that any blow to or laceration of the scalp arteries renders them more liable to the painful dilatation that gives rise to post-traumatic migraine. The area of pain may be limited to a particular vessel in the forehead, temple, or back of the head in the part that was struck at the time of the injury. Sometimes a scar may traverse one of the major scalp arteries. Jabbing pains may also be felt at the site of a scar where nerves have been involved in the scar tissue. An operation to tie off and cut the affected artery (and nerve as well, if it is also involved) often gives relief. Otherwise, the treatment is the same as for migraine. Jabbing nerve pains usually respond well to medication with carbamazepine.

In addition to the migrainous pattern of headache, there is another form of vascular headache that may be caused by dilatation of the intracranial vessels and aggravated further by vasodilator agents such as histamine. It is frequently found in conjunction with muscle-contraction headaches after head injury and is exacerbated by exertion.

Whiplash Injury

The dramatic term "whiplash injury" conjures up a vision of the patient's neck being cracked like a whip—imagery more vivid than is usually warranted by the circumstances. The use of the term may be enough to make the patient retract the neck like a tortoise, causing the neck muscles to contract continuously. This is a potent cause of headache in its own right. In any accident where the body is stabilized and the head is free to move, some degree of whiplash takes place. The classic example is the driver in a stationary car that is hit in the rear by another vehicle. The front car is pushed forward, the driver's back is pressed against the seat, and the head is forced backward. The reverse situation may occur when the driver of the moving car is wearing a seat belt that restrains the body at the moment when the car collides with another, so that the head flexes violently forward on the neck.

Immediately after such a collision the neck may feel stiff and sore, and pain may occur in the back of the head. Mercifully, these symptoms usually disappear after a few days of discomfort and all is well again. When pain persists, the condition is often difficult to assess objectively, as X rays of the neck usually show no recent abnormality, and judgment must be made entirely on clinical grounds. Pain may radiate down to the shoulders and arms or up to the back of the head and even to the forehead. There may be local tenderness in the neck or the back of the skull. The pain can be derived from a displacement of part of the substance of a disk that lies between two vertebral bodies as a shock absorber (Figures 2.1, 10.3). Pain can also arise from the interpedicular joints of the vertebrae (Figure 10.3), from the ligaments and soft tissues of the neck, or from stretching of nerve roots.

The condition may be treated by injecting local anesthetic agents and hydrocortisone or long-acting steroids into the tender areas. It may also require immobilizing the neck with a plastic collar. The application of local heat and traction to the neck by a physiotherapist is often helpful. There are those who advocate manipulation of the neck, but this should be done only by professionals, for there is potential danger that the disk substance may be forced onto the spinal cord. This can cause complete paralysis of the legs, severe weakness of the arms, and loss of bladder and bowel function.

Dr. James Cyriax of St. Thomas's Hospital, London, who had long practiced manipulation of the neck, stressed that it should be done without any anesthesia (26). The patient should lie on the back with the head over the end of a bed, so that traction can be exerted on the neck in the extended position while the manipulation is in progress. With these precautions, he had never seen any untoward effect and achieved some remarkably beneficial results.

In some cases, the factor of compensation neurosis or even frankly hysterical behavior can add to the problem. I recall one patient who walked normally while wearing a surgical collar. On every occasion when the collar was removed, he underwent weird gyrations, flailing his arms and legs. Eventually he fell to the floor. A collar may be good treatment for a while, but it is not essential for maintaining an upright posture and should not be permanently allowed to take the place of the neck muscles.

Muscular Contraction

Dr. Harold Wolff examined a group of sixty-three patients with chronic post-traumatic headache and recorded the electrical activity in the muscles of the scalp and neck (114). He found that the muscles were continuously active in three-quarters of the patients for the duration of their headache. In twenty-eight of the thirty-seven people examined during a headache, the muscle activity was greatest at the site of the headache. This does not mean that excessive muscle contraction is necessarily the cause of the headache, but it can be an important factor, since mental and physical relaxation may reduce or eliminate the headache. This process was discussed in greater detail in chapter 8.

The quality of muscle-contraction headache is usually a dull pressure sensation or tightness in the head. The pressure is fairly continuous but fluctuates in intensity, occasionally flaring up to a more painful throbbing when vascular dilatation is superimposed. The sufferers are usually tense, anxious, fretful, and often depressed. They may also be resentful about the accident, the legal implications, and possibly the treatment they have or have not received from their doctors. All of this may be reinforced if they are referred from doctor to doctor for opinions. The treatment is similar to that for tension headache (described in chapter 8), but it depends for its success on a doctor taking a personal and sustained interest in the patient's welfare.

Tumor and Trauma

Head injuries are very common, and brain tumors are rare. Nevertheless, an association has been drawn between head injury and the later development, up to thirty years afterward, of a meningioma, a benign tumor growing from the membranes of the skull. The association was first noted by the famous neurosurgeon Dr. Harvey Cushing of Johns Hopkins Hospital, Baltimore; in 30 percent of his three hundred patients with meningioma, the tumor developed at the site of previous damage to the skull. This contention is hard to prove statistically, but it has been supported by the experience of many authors, including Sir Francis Walshe, who concluded, "The perpetually open mind is not an effective instrument of thought, and may too easily become a euphemism for the mind closed to the lessons of experience" (111).

Compensation and Litigation

If the persistence of symptoms after head injury were due to a conscious or subconscious desire for financial gain, it might be assumed that they would be present less often in those whose injury was not compensable and would disappear once the case was settled in the patient's favor. Neither of these suppositions is invariably correct. Cynics used to say that the cure for the post-traumatic syndrome is to insert gold into the palm of the hand. But is this the cure? Dr. John Balla and Dr. S. Moraitis from Melbourne followed up the cases of eighty-two patients of Greek extraction after they had been in industrial or traffic accidents that caused injuries to their necks and backs. Forty-one of them complained of bilateral headaches radiating up from the neck like a pressure sensation. Although original injuries were mild and many of the patients' symptoms were considered to have a psychological basis, the correlation between early settlement of the legal case and return to work was not high. At the time of settlement, forty had already gone back to work and eleven did so shortly afterward. But thirty-one patients continued to have symptoms that prevented them from working, even after the case had been decided and financial compensation awarded.

That symptoms disappear in some patients who return to work before settlement of claims and persist in others after compensation has been agreed upon should not disguise the fact that some patients do lack any motivation to return to work and that others have quite bizarre psychological reactions toward their injury and its legal aspects.

Neurotic or Organic?

Controversy still rages over the degree to which symptoms that follow head injury are determined by the medicolegal aspects, by a psychological reaction to injury, or by some subtle organic change. Some of the symptoms of anxiety and depression following head injury have already been mentioned. Schizophrenia with paranoid ideas, hysterical conversion reactions, and hypochondriasis may also be precipitated by head injury (37).

One of my own patients underwent a complete personality change after being knocked unconscious while working in a mine. His workmates mistakenly elected to drive him to the nearest hospital by car, although he was still unconscious. He was supported in the sitting position, which reduced the blood supply to his concussed brain. After apparent physical recovery from his injury, he changed from being a reliable, steady worker to a shiftless, evasive character with grossly hysterical behavior. He stated that he was unable to feel pain and demonstrated this by stubbing out cigarette butts on his arm or leg. Pathological changes have been observed in nerve cells as a result of brain concussion, and it seems reasonable to assume that in some patients these could account for an alteration in personality. Certainly some patients can never perform again at their previous level.

Whether minute changes in the structure of brain cells also play a part in the symptoms of anxiety and depression so frequent after head injury remains open to question. The self-employed return to work earlier, on the average, than those who are employed by others. This may be a question of motivation, but could also be related to the greater physical exertion required of employees in many industries, especially semiskilled workers and laborers—exertion that may make certain persistent symptoms intolerable.

There is good evidence that the giddiness that commonly follows head injury is caused by damage to that part of the inner ear concerned with the sense of balance. It may well be that many of the other symptoms have their basis in some form of damage that we are unable to detect by present methods. This is the view put forward by Dr. Alex R. Taylor, a neurosurgeon from Belfast in Northern Ireland. He says, "Prima facie, it seems strange that 66 percent of the head-injured, necessarily a random sample of the population, should be afflicted with neuroticism or excessive cupidity while most of the victims of limb, abdominal, or thoracic injury escape these stigmata. The evidence for neuroticism should be carefully examined" (109).

On the other side of the ledger, the late Professor Henry Miller of Newcastle-upon-Tyne presented a case for the multitude of symptoms being a purely psychological reaction to the accident (80). He found that the majority of his patients lost their symptoms after legal settlement. Only two out of fifty unselected patients were still disabled two years after settlement. The most that the other patients could muster were a few trivial, residual symptoms, such as "a queer feeling as I turn on the vacuum cleaner" and "some nervousness on overtaking in traffic." Miller concludes: "It seems clear that accident neurosis is not a function of the accident itself, but of the setting in which this occurred. In my opinion it is not a result of the accident but a concomitant of the compensation situation and a manifestation of the hope of financial gain." He makes a point that emphasizes the paradox in the treatment of this problem: "Doctor and lawyer are sometimes at cross-purposes over the question of settlement, the lawyer insisting that there should be no settlement without clinical finality, the doctor that there can be no clinical finality without settlement."

A Balanced View

Arguments have been presented for both sides of the case— are the symptoms psychological or organic? Considering that the mind is the product of the brain, the gap between these arguments may be narrowed.

We recognize extracranial vascular headaches similar to migraine resulting from damage to scalp vessels, and a less clearly defined intracranial vascular headache that may be

made worse by exertion. This suggests that the very fact of a
sudden acceleration or deceleration of the head may be sufficient to render cranial blood vessels more susceptible to painful
dilatation. We recognize aching in the back of the head as related to disturbance of the upper neck. We concede that excessive muscle contraction may play a part in maintaining the
headache pattern after the initial structural damage has
subsided.

The anxiety and depression that accompany muscle contraction seems to be initially related to the accident, although
litigation worries may later aggravate the situation. Patients
are naturally fearful that they will never be quite the same as
before and that their capacity for work may be impaired. There
is also the dread of another accident. I was once the victim of
an explosion that caused extensive burns to my face and arm,
and I well recall that my responses to any sudden sound were
exaggerated for some weeks or months afterward. An extreme
example of this fear was described by John Ellard, a psychiatrist at the Northside Clinic, Sydney. A woman who had been
involved in an automobile accident could tolerate being driven
by her husband only if she could huddle under a rug on the
floor in the back of the car drinking brandy. Problems like this
require sympathetic understanding and psychotherapy.

Finally, there are always those who regard an accident as a
gift from the gods, a ticket in a lottery that may win them a
substantial prize if they can hang on to the ticket long enough.

It requires an unbiased approach on the part of the doctor, a
careful assessment of each patient's personality and headache
pattern, and a considerable degree of skill to ensure that justice
serves the patient's legal claim and that treatment is appropriate to the variety of headache.

14

YOU AND
YOUR DOCTOR

Which Doctor?

The most important ally a headache patient can have is a sympathetic general practitioner who knows the patient, his or her family, and his or her problems as a basis for coming to grips with the headache itself. This presupposes that the family doctor has sufficient time to spend with patients who require it and is familiar with the advances that have been made in the classification, diagnosis, and treatment of headaches over recent years. It may seem that this is looking for perfection and yet this sort of understanding and guidance can still be found in this hurried age. I recommend that the patient first consult a general practitioner, because no end of trouble can arise from patients shuttling from one specialist to another without being referred by their family doctor. The general practitioner can correlate reports from specialists and apply their findings to the best advantage. It is conceivable that a patient with headache could consult an eye doctor who prescribes glasses, an ear, nose, and throat doctor who fixes up his or her sinus trouble, followed by an orthopedic surgeon who treats a cervical disk disturbance, and so on, while the headache continues unabated. Fortunately, this is not very likely because most specialists realize immediately whether a problem lies within their province. However, the family general practitioner is in the best position to assess whether one of these specialists or a general physician, neurologist, or psychiatrist would be of the most assistance in each individual case. It may well be that your G.P. takes a particular interest in headache problems and can set you on the right road without the need to see a consultant. The important principle is that there must be one doctor who is *your* doctor, who has your interests at heart.

Please Have Your Symptoms Ready

There is a story that a frazzled general practitioner placed a sign in the waiting room saying, "Please have your symptoms ready." Examinations are greatly facilitated if patients have organized their thoughts and are ready to answer the physician's questions. If the doctor asks how long you have had your headache, he or she is after an approximation and is not usually concerned about the precise day, week, or month. I recommend making brief notes of the salient features so that the pattern of headache becomes clear to you and your doctor. It is helpful if you tell the doctor the symptoms that concern you, their duration, their pattern of recurrence, and what factors alter them. After this, the doctor will probably want certain other specific information. Every doctor has a slightly different approach. Some prefer to ask leading questions throughout. Others like patients to tell the story in their own words. Most combine the two methods. Whatever the approach, there is an obvious advantage if you have your thoughts marshaled before the consultation begins.

The Pattern of Headache

Throughout this book the emphasis has been on diagnosis from the clinical history. Only rarely are special tests required to confirm or deny a certain hypothesis. If the story is presented clearly, the diagnosis will usually become evident as it progresses. Some basic information is required, and the following headings will help you to "have your symptoms ready."

How long have you suffered from headache? Days, weeks, months, or years?

How often does the headache recur? Once a year, once a month, several times a week, or daily?

How long does the headache last? Minutes, hours, or days? Please correlate this with the preceding question. Patients sometimes say that they have, say, three headaches a week, each lasting three days, when what they mean is that the one weekly headache lasts for three days and they then have a break for three or four days before the next one starts.

Is there any pattern to the recurrence of the headache? Does it go away for months at a time, then return in the manner of cluster headache? Has it increased in frequency or changed its pattern lately? Are there two or more varieties of headache that should be analyzed separately? For example, migraine and tension headache may coexist, so that the daily dull ache caused by muscle contraction may be punctuated by more severe episodes of migraine.

What area of the head is affected? Both sides or one side only? Right or left or alternating? Is it just one part of the head (forehead, temple, or the back of the head), or is it all over the head? Does it radiate down the neck or elsewhere?

What is the quality of the pain? Is it constant or fluctuating, dull or severe? Does it throb (intensify with each beat of the pulse)?

How does it start? Is the headache present on waking in the morning, or does it waken you from sleep in the middle of the night? Does it come on during the day? If so, are there any warning symptoms, such as visual or other sensory disturbances or a change of mood?

What are the associated features? Do you feel nauseated, vomit, or pass loose bowel movements? Does light hurt your eyes, or does noise worry you? This list of questions could be extended almost indefinitely by referring to the sections dealing with each variety of headache.

Are there any precipitating factors? Does the headache come on at moments of emotional disturbance or nervous tension or at times of relaxation, such as weekends? Does it recur at any particular phase of the menstrual cycle? Is it related to physical exercise, to the taking of certain foods or alcohol, or any other known factors?

Are there any aggravating factors? Is the headache made

worse by sudden movement of the head or neck? Is it worse on coughing, sneezing, or straining? Is it worse when standing or when lying down?

Are there any relieving factors? Do hot or cold packs or any other physical measures help? Will the headache go away if you lie down and sleep? Is it eased by ordinary analgesics such as aspirin, acetophenetidin (phenacetin), acetaminophen (paracetamol; Tylenol), or by stronger tablets containing codeine? Does it ever require injections given by your doctor?

Have you had any other treatment for an acute attack of headache? What were they, and did they stop the headache?

Have you had regular medication of any sort in an attempt to prevent the headache completely? If so, what was the result?

Have you had any other treatment—manipulation of the neck, physiotherapy, acupuncture, or psychotherapy?

Helping Your Doctor

Once your doctor has a clear and concise picture of your type of headache, he or she will probably ask about your general health, your past health (with particular reference to head injuries), your family history (with emphasis on headache of any sort), and your personal background. Be honest in your description of smoking habits, alcohol, and your use of any other drugs. Discuss frankly any fear or anxiety that is troubling you, and do not hesitate to bring up sexual problems if there are any. What may seem to be a very grave, embarrassing, or insuperable problem to you could well be one your doctor has encountered many times before and that may be overcome with the right advice. If you have some particular worry you wish to discuss, bring it up early in the interview so there is time to go into it.

Be honest with yourself and with your doctor about any symptoms of depression, as these may be responsible for daily headaches or can develop as a reaction to frequent headache. In either event, the vicious cycle can often be broken by the relief of depression, and there are now many ways of doing this pharmacologically as well as psychologically.

You can help your doctor by presenting your symptoms logically and briefly and by replying as clearly as possible to his or her questions. Since the doctor's diagnosis depends upon an analysis of the history you give, the whole examination is a collaborative venture. Ideally, you know and have confidence in your doctor. Your doctor respects you as an individual and is anxious to help you. This is a solid basis on which to build.

Helping Yourself

After reading this book you should have a sound idea of the principles of headache, its diagnosis, and its treatment. It is intended to help in interpreting and carrying out your doctor's advice.

If your headaches continue after trying a particular form of treatment, you should not consult a different doctor immediately. Stay with the first doctor so that he or she can proceed with various treatments in regular sequence. If you switch to another doctor, the second doctor will probably have to start at the same point as the first and may even prescribe the same treatment unless you explain that you responded poorly to it.

If your own doctor is in doubt about the diagnosis or treatment, he or she can refer you to the most appropriate specialist. No matter how much experience one has, another point of view and a fresh assessment of the case are always welcome. I greatly appreciate the opinion of my colleagues on many different neurological problems. There are occasions when a newly graduated doctor or a medical student may suddenly hit on something that has escaped those with greater experience and may place the diagnostic key within one's grasp. If this is the case, how much more often must a doctor in the most difficult of all specialties, general practice, be glad of another's opinion.

One final point. If treatment is prescribed, please give it a fair trial. There is nothing more frustrating than agreeing on a course of action that is never carried out or prescribing a medication that is never taken. The success of any treatment depends on your own understanding and cooperation as well as your doctor's knowledge and ability.

Freedom from Headache

There are some forms of headache that can be cured completely. Most can be helped considerably. For the common condition of tension headache, there is much that can be done by the individual. The treatment depends on the patient as much as the doctor. The way of life and the mental approach to its problems are as important as medication. There are few forms of headache that will respond to one treatment and one treatment only. Most have many facets, each of which must be examined. With migraine as with cluster headache, all the clues seem to be at hand to solve the mystery. I feel optimistic that the next ten years will bring us closer to a solution of these problems. Even if the complete answer is not obtained, advances in knowledge as great as those of the last ten years will enable treatment to become still more effective, until at last the doctor can offer every patient his or her natural right—freedom from headache.

Thomas Willis in the seventeenth century said, "It has become a proverb as a sign of a most rare and admirable thing, 'that his head did never ake.' "

GLOSSARY

Adrenal glands. Glands situated above the kidneys. The central part (medulla) secretes epinephrine (adrenaline) and norepinephrine (noradrenaline). Both amines circulate in the bloodstream and constrict the cranial arteries, as well as increasing blood pressure and pulse rate. The outer part of the gland (cortex) produces cortisone.

Air encephalography. An X-ray technique involving the insertion of about 30 milliliters of air into the cerebrospinal fluid to outline the ventricles and other fluid-containing canals in and around the brain. Rarely used since the advent of CT scanning.

Alpha rhythm. The dominant brain rhythm recorded in a normal electroencephalogram, usually eight to ten per second.

Amitriptyline. An antidepressant agent useful in managing tension headache and other types of chronic pain.

Amyl nitrite. A vasodilator substance occasionally used in managing angina pectoris and in reducing the spasm of vessels in some cases of migraine.

Analgesics. Substances that relieve pain, such as aspirin.

Aneurysm. A localized dilatation of an artery in which the wall is weaker than a normal artery and may leak to cause subarachnoid hemorrhage.

Angiogram, arteriogram. A specialized X-ray technique in which a radio-opaque dye is injected into an artery to demonstrate whether the blood vessels are normal. See also Digital subtraction angiography.

Angioma, arteriovenous malformation. An abnormal collection of blood vessels, analogous to a red birthmark, in which blood passes rapidly from arteries to veins.

Aqueduct. A channel in the brain that conveys cerebrospinal fluid from the third to the fourth ventricle.

Arachnoid. A delicate membrane that surrounds the brain and spinal cord and contains the cerebrospinal fluid.

Atheroma. A fatty deposit in the arterial wall that is a common cause of stroke and coronary occlusion.

Basilar artery. An artery formed by the junction of the two vertebral arteries, which supplies the brain stem. It then divides to form two posterior cerebral arteries that supply the visual cortex.

Basilar migraine. A form of migraine in which the branches of the basilar artery are affected, causing symptoms such as giddiness, loss of balance, faintness, and visual disturbances.

Beta-blockers. Drugs, such as propranolol, that block the action of norepinephrine on beta-receptors responsible for dilating blood vessels and bronchi as well as increasing heart rate. Beta-blockers thus slow heart rate and prevent dilatation of blood vessels and bronchi. Some drugs have a relatively selective effect on the heart and vessels.

Biofeedback. A technique that gives information to subjects about a bodily function to help them exert control over that function. For example, the degree of muscle contraction can be signaled by the intensity of a sound and thus helps the subject relax that muscle.

Bradykinin. A peptide released in inflammatory processes, causing dilatation of blood vessels.

Brain stem. A part of the hindbrain resembling a stem or stalk between the midbrain and spinal cord. It contains the nuclei of most of the cranial nerves as well as vital centers concerned with breathing and maintaining blood pressure.

Calcium-channel blockers. Drugs that prevent calcium uptake by the muscular wall of blood vessels, thereby preventing the vessels from constricting.

Carbamazepine. An anticonvulsant drug that reduces the jabbing pains of tic douloureux (trade name Tegretol).

Carcinoid. A tumor of the gastrointestinal tract that secretes serotonin.

Carotid arteries. Large arteries that course through the neck to supply the greater part of the brain through their anterior and middle cerebral branches.

Cerebrospinal fluid. A clear liquid manufactured by the choroid plexuses in the ventricles of the brain, which circulates around the brain and helps to support and protect it.

Cervical migraine. A type of headache, with characteristics similar to basilar migraine, said to be caused by spurs of bone compressing the vertebral arteries in their course through the cervical spine.

Cervical spine. The bones (vertebrae) of the neck that enclose the spinal cord. The vertebral arteries lie in a canal within the side projections of the bones.

Choroid plexuses. Capillary networks in the ventricles of the brain that form the cerebrospinal fluid.

Chronic paroxysmal hemicrania (CPH). A variation of cluster headache with frequent, brief episodes of pain recurring during each twenty-four-hour period.

Ciliary neuralgia. An old name for cluster headache.

Cluster headache. A type of headache recurring in bouts or clusters. Also called migrainous neuralgia or Horton's histaminic cephalgia.

Computerized transverse axial tomography (CT or CAT scanning). A new method of X-ray localization of intracranial structures. A thin beam of X rays scans the head in a series of planes. Minute differences in the absorption of the rays are calculated by computer and displayed as a pictorial representation of the intracranial contents in each plane.

Cortisone. A steroid hormone made by the cortex of the adrenal glands. Synthetic forms of this hormone are used in treatment.

Costen's syndrome. Pain radiating over the face from the hinge joint of the jaw in front of the ear, commonly caused by an imbalanced bite and jaw-clenching. Also called temporomandibular joint (TMJ) dysfunction.

Cranial nerves. Twelve pairs arising from or entering the brain, each pair concerned with special functions such as the sense of smell (1), vision (2), eye movements (3, 4, 6), facial sensations and jaw movements (5), facial movement (7), hearing (8), swallowing and speech (9, 10), head-turning (11), and tongue movement (12).

Cyproheptadine. An agent used in the prevention of migraine.

Diazepam. A tranquilizing, anticonvulsant, and muscle-relaxing agent (trade name Valium).

Digital subtraction angiography. A computerized technique that enhances the quality of angiograms. The contrast medium may be injected into an artery or a vein.

Diuretic.   An agent that reduces the amount of body fluid by promoting the excretion of salt and water in the urine.

Dura.   A firm membrane lining the inner side of the skull.

Edema.   Swelling of a tissue caused by excessive fluid in the cells or surrounding tissues.

Electroencephalogram (EEG).   A recording of the electrical activity arising from the brain.

Encephalitis.   A viral infection of the brain.

Endorphins.   Endogenous morphinelike substances. See Opioids.

Enkephalins.   Chemical transmitters employed by the body's pain-control system. See Opioids.

Epinephrine (adrenaline).   See Adrenal glands.

Ergotamine tartrate.   A chemical agent derived from ergot that constricts the arteries of the scalp and is used for this purpose in treating migraine.

Estrogen.   A female hormone, the blood level of which falls just before menstruation and is a trigger factor for premenstrual migraine.

Fenemates.   Nonsteroidal anti-inflammatory drugs that may be useful in aborting acute attacks of migraine.

GABA.   Gamma aminobutyric acid. An inhibitory transmitter that is thought to diminish the passage of pain impulses in the central nervous system.

Glaucoma.   Increased pressure within the eyeball.

Glial cells.   Connective tissue cells that lie between the nerve cells of the brain and help to nourish them.

Glioma.   A tumor arising from glial cells.

Glossopharyngeal nerve.   The ninth cranial nerve that supplies sensation to part of the ear and the back of the throat as well as innervating muscles concerned with swallowing.

Glossopharyngeal neuralgia.   Painful jabs of pain in the ear and throat caused by irritation of the glossopharyngeal nerve.

Hemicrania.   An ache involving one-half of the head only.

Hemiplegic migraine.   A form of migraine, commonly hereditary, in which one-half of the body becomes weak.

Heparin.   An anticlotting agent contained in body mast cells.

Herpes zoster.   Shingles. A red rash with blisters developing in the distribution of nerve roots, sometimes followed by pain (postherpetic neuralgia).

Histamine.   An amine contained in mast cells and other tissues that is released in allergic reactions and causes dilatation of cranial blood vessels.

Horton's histaminic cephalgia.   See Cluster headache.

Hydrocephalus.   Increased intracranial pressure caused by obstruction to the flow of cerebrospinal fluid or failure of its absorption.

Ice-cream headache.   Transient head pain on swallowing cold food or drink.

Ice-pick pains.   Jabbing pains in the head, commonly associated with migraine or tension headache.

Indomethacin.   An inhibitor of prostaglandin formation used in the treatment of arthritis and that has also been employed in ice-pick pains, exertional headache, and chronic paroxysmal hemicrania. It can cause a continuous dull headache as a side effect (trade name Indocin).

Isotope scanning.   The use of radioactive isotopes to detect changes in vascularity of tissues. The usual form of brain scanning is injecting the isotope into a vein and recording the isotope passing up the neck vessels into the brain by a gamma camera (dynamic scanning). Later recordings are taken once the isotope is distributed in the brain tissue (static scanning).

Locus ceruleus.   A collection of cells containing norepinephrine and melanin lying in the brain stem. Melanin gives the nucleus a blue-black appearance to the naked eye, hence the name. It has diffuse connections that play a part in regulating cortical activity and the pain-control system.

Lumbar puncture.   The insertion of a fine needle through the skin of the back (lumbar region) into the fluid-containing sac below the lower end of the spinal cord. The procedure is done under local anesthesia to obtain a sample of the cerebrospinal fluid for analysis, or to inject air or dye for specialized X rays.

Magnetic resonance imaging.   See Nuclear magnetic resonance.

Mast cells.   Cells containing granules of histamine and heparin that surround scalp arteries.

Melanoma.   A malignant mole.

Meninges.   Membranes of the brain. The dura lines the inner side of the skull, the arachnoid contains the cerebrospinal fluid, and the pia covers the brain surface.

Meningioma.   A tumor arising from the meninges.

Meningism.   Irritation of the meninges without inflammation.

Meningitis.   Inflammation of the meninges, usually caused by bacteria.

Meningoencephalitis.   Inflammation of the meninges and brain, usually caused by a virus.

Methysergide. A pharmaceutical agent used in the prevention of migraine (trade names Sansert, Deseril).

Midbrain. Region of the brain between the cerebral hemispheres and the brain stem, containing the area responsible for maintaining consciousness.

Monoamine oxidase (MAO). An enzyme that breaks down monoamines such as serotonin, epinephrine, and norepinephrine. Another type of MAO breaks down phenylethylamine, which is found in chocolate. Drugs that inhibit MAO are used in the treatment of depression as well as migraine.

Myalgia. Muscle pain.

Neuralgia. Pain arising from inflammation or compression of nerves.

Neurotransmitter. A chemical agent liberated by a nerve terminal to excite or inhibit other nerve cells with which it comes in contact. Examples are serotonin, norepinephrine, GABA.

Norepinephrine. See Adrenal glands.

Nuclear magnetic resonance. A technique for obtaining an image of the brain or other parts of the body by applying a magnetic field.

Ophthalmoplegic migraine. Migraine headache associated with double vision caused by weakness of the eye muscles.

Opioids. Naturally occurring substances that have an effect in the body similar to derivatives of opium, such as morphine. Also called endorphins.

Papilledema. Swelling of the optic nerve head in the eye, which can be seen with an ophthalmoscope and is one sign of raised intracranial pressure.

Phenylethylamine. A amine present in chocolate that has been implicated as a possible trigger for migraine.

Pheochromocytoma. A tumor of the adrenal gland producing epinephrine and norepinephrine that may be responsible for raising blood pressure.

Photophobia. Aversion to light.

Pia. The inner of the three brain membranes (meninges).

Pizotifen, pizotylene. An agent used in the prevention of migraine (trade name Sandomigran).

Positron emission tomography (PET scanning). A technique whereby substances like glucose are attached to (labeled with) a positron-emitting isotope. Pictures like CT scans then show where the substance is taken up by the brain and can indicate the rate at which it is being used up in the brain.

Postherpetic neuralgia. Pain following herpes zoster (shingles).

Progesterone. A female hormone that becomes elevated in the blood during the second half of the menstrual cycle and during pregnancy.

Prostaglandins. A series of complex fatty acids that affect blood vessels, among other actions. Originally named because of their association with the prostate gland.

Raphe nuclei. Midline nuclei of the brain stem that contain serotonin and play a part in the pain-control system, as well as sending fibers to the cerebral cortex.

REM sleep. Rapid-eye-movement phase of sleep. A periodic lightened level of sleep in which eye movement occurs.

Serotonin. An amine manufactured in the intestinal wall and carried in blood platelets, from which it may be released to affect blood vessels. Also found in nerve cells and other tissues.

Steroids. A group of substances that includes cortisone. The term steroids is used loosely for natural and synthetic forms of cortisone used in treatment.

Subarachnoid hemorrhage. Bleeding into the cerebrospinal fluid, contained in the space beneath the arachnoid membrane.

Subdural hematoma. Bleeding into the space outside the arachnoid membrane but beneath the dura.

Substance P. A peptide neurotransmitter that plays a part in dilatation of blood vessels and in the conduction of pain impulses.

Suprachiasmatic nucleus. A collection of nerve cells situated above the chiasm (crossing of optic nerve fibers) and responsible for setting circadian (daily) rhythms such as sleep.

Temporal arteritis. Inflammation of the temporal arteries in the scalp, which may also affect other vessels of the scalp, brain, and eye.

Thermocoagulation. Applying heat to an area to cause partial destruction. Used to damage nerve cells in the trigeminal ganglion to prevent the pain of tic douloureux.

Thermography. The measurement of heat given off from an object by an infrared detector.

Tic douloureux. Severe jabbing pain caused by irritation of the trigeminal nerve. Also called trigeminal neuralgia.

Tomography. An X-ray beam focused on a particular layer or plane in order to display it clearly.

Transmitter. See Neurotransmitter.

Trauma. Injury.

Trigeminal nerve. The nerve supplying sensation to the face. It has three divisions, hence the name trigeminal ("three born at once").

Trigeminal neuralgia. See Tic douloureux.

Tyramine. An amine present in some foods that is thought to be a trigger factor in some forms of migraine.

Vasoactive intestinal polypeptide (VIP). A peptide neurotransmitter first found in the intestine, hence its name. It dilates blood vessels and probably has additional actions in the central nervous system.

Vasomotor rhinitis. Blockage of the nostrils by swollen blood vessels in the mucous membrane of the nose.

Ventricles. Canals within the brain containing the cerebrospinal fluid. There are paired lateral ventricles that open into the third ventricle, from which the fluid passes to the fourth ventricle through the aqueduct.

Ventriculography. Demonstration of the size and position of the ventricles by an X-ray technique that involves injecting air or a radio-opaque substance into them.

Vertebral arteries. Arteries ascending in a canal within the neck vertebrae that unite to form the basilar artery.

Vertebrobasilar insufficiency. Failure of blood flow through the vertebral and basilar arteries, causing symptoms similar to basilar migraine.

Vertigo. Giddiness, a sense of movement of the head in relation to the environment or vice versa.

REFERENCES

(1) Adams, F. *The Seven Books of Paulus Aegineta.* London: Sydenham Society, 1844.

(2) Adams, F. *The Extant Works of Aretaeus, the Cappadocian.* London: Sydenham Society, 1841.

(3) Adams, F. *The Genuine Works of Hippocrates.* Baltimore: Williams & Wilkins, 1939.

(4) Anderson, B., Jr.; Heyman, A.; Whalen, R. E.; and Saltzmann, H. A. Migraine-like phenomena after decompression from hyperbaric environment. *Neurology* (Minneapolis) 15:1035, 1965.

(5) Anthony, M.; Hinterberger, H.; and Lance, J. W. The possible relationship of serotonin to the migraine syndrome, in *Research and Clinical Studies in Headache*, Vol. 2. New York & Basel: Karger, 1968, p. 29.

(6) Anthony, M., and Lance, J. W. Monoamine oxidase inhibition in the treatment of migraine. *Archives of Neurology* 21:263, 1969.

(7) Anthony, M., and Lance, J. W. Histamine and serotonin in cluster headache. *Archives of Neurology* 25:225, 1971.

(8) Balla, J. I., and Moraitis, S. Knights in armour: A follow-up study of injuries after legal settlement. *Medical Journal of Australia* 2:355, 1970.

(9) Basbaum, A. I., and Fields, H. L. Endogenous pain control mechanisms: Review and hypothesis. *Annals of Neurology* 4:451, 1978.

(10) Bennett, D. R.; Feunning, S. I.; Sullivan, G.; and Weber, J. Migraine precipitated by head trauma in athletes. *American Journal of Sports Medicine* 8:202, 1980.

(11) Benson, H.; Klemchuk, H. P.; and Graham, J. R. The usefulness of the relaxation response in the therapy of headache. *Headache* 14:49, 1974.

(12) Bickerstaff, E. R. Impairment of consciousness in migraine. *Lancet* 2:1057, 1961.

(13) Bille, B. Migraine in school-children. *Acta Paediatrica* (Stockholm) 51(supplement 136):1, 1962.

(14) Bille, B. Migraine in childhood and its prognosis. *Cephalalgia* 1:71, 1981.

(15) Blau, J. N., and Cumings, J. N. Method of precipitating and preventing some migraine attacks. *British Medical Journal* 2:1242, 1966.

(16) Blau, J. N., and Pyke, D. A. Effect of diabetes on migraine. *Lancet* 2:241, 1970.

(17) Bogduk, N. The anatomy of occipital neuralgia. *Clinical and Experimental Neurology* 17:167, 1980.

(18) Brenner, C.; Friedman, Arnold P.; Merritt, H. H.; and Denny-Brown, D. E. Post-traumatic headache. *Journal of Neurosurgery* 6:379, 1944.

(19) Brewis, M.; Poskanzer, D. C.; Rolland, C.; and Miller, H. Neurological disease in an English city. *Acta Neurologica Scandinavica* 42(supplement 24):1, 1963.

(20) Brindley, G. S., and Lewin, B. S. The sensations produced by electrical stimulation of the visual cortex. *Journal of Physiology* 196:479, 1968.

(21) Broch, A.; Hørven, I.; Nornes, H.; Sjaastad, O.; and Tønjum, A. Studies on cerebral and ocular circulation in a patient with cluster headache. *Headache* 10:1, 1970.

(22) Cleland, J., and Southcott, R. V. Hypervitaminosis A in the Antarctic in the Australasian Antarctic expedition of 1911–1914: A possible explanation of the illnesses of Mertz and Mawson. *Medical Journal of Australia* 1:1337, 1969.

(23) Costen, J. B. A syndrome of ear and sinus symptoms dependent upon disturbed function of the temporomandibular joint. *Annals of Otology, Rhinology and Laryngology* 43: 1, 1934.

(24) Critchley, M. Migraine from Cappadocia to Queen Square, in *Background to Migraine*, Vol. 1. London: Heinemann, 1967, p. 28.

(25) Cull, R. E. Barometric pressure and other factors in migraine. *Headache* 21:102, 1981.

(26) Cyriax, J. *Textbook of Orthopaedic Medicine*, Vol. 1. London: Cassell, 1962.

(27) Dalsgaard-Nielsen, T. Some aspects of the epidemiology of migraine in Denmark, in *Kliniske Aspekter i Migraeneforskningen*. Copenhagen: Nordlundes Bogtrykkeri, 1970, p. 18.

(28) Dexter, J. D., and Weitzman, E. D. The relationship of nocturnal headaches to sleep stage patterns. *Neurology* (Minneapolis) 20:513, 1970.

(29) Drake, D. *A Systematic Treatise, Historical, Epidemiological and Practical, on the Principal Diseases of the Interior Valley on North America, as May Appear in the Caucasian, African and Indian and Esquimaux Varieties of Its Population.* Cincinnati: W. B. Smith & Co., 1850.

(30) Drummond, P. D.; Gonski, A.; and Lance, J. W. Facial flushing after thermocoagulation of the Gasserian ganglion. *Journal of Neurology, Neurosurgery and Psychiatry* 46:32, 1983.

(31) Drummond, P. D., and Lance, J. W. Extracranial vascular changes and the source of pain in migraine headache. *Annals of Neurology* 13:32, 1983.

(32) Drummond, P. D., and Lance, J. W. Clinical diagnosis and computer analysis of headache symptoms. *Journal of Neurology, Neurosurgery and Psychiatry* 47:128, 1984.

(33) Drummond, P. D., and Lance, J. W. Neurovascular disturbances in headache patients. *Clinical and Experimental Neurology* 20:93, 1984.

(34) Drummond, P. D., and Lance, J. W. Thermographic changes in cluster headache. *Neurology* (Cleveland) 34:1292, 1984.

(35) Egger, J.; Carter, C. M.; Wilson, J.; Turner, M. W.; and Southill, J. F. Is migraine food allergy? A double-blind controlled trial of oligoantigenic diet treatment. *Lancet* 2:865, 1983.

(36) Ekbom, K. Clinical aspects of cluster headache. *Headache* 13:176, 1974.

(37) Ellard, J. Psychological reactions to compensable injury. *Medical Journal of Australia* 2:349, 1970.

(38) Elliott, F. A. Treatment of herpes zoster with high doses of prednisone. *Lancet* 2:610, 1964.

(39) Engel, G. L.; Ferris, E. B.; and Romano, J. Focal electroencephalographic changes during the scotomas of migraine. *American Journal of Medical Science* 209:650, 1945.

(40) Friedman, A. P. The (infinite) variety of migraine: Sandoz Foundation lecture, in *Background to Migraine*. Third Migraine Symposium. London: Heinemann, 1970, p. 165.

(41) Friedman, A. P. The headache in history, literature and legend. *Bulletin of the New York Academy of Medicine* 48:661, 1972.

(42) Goadsby, P. J.; Lambert, G. A.; and Lance, J. W. Differential effects on the internal and external carotid circulation of the monkey evoked by locus coeruleus stimulation. *Brain Research* 249:247, 1982.

(43) Goadsby, P. J., and Macdonald, G. J. Extracranial vasodilatation mediated by VIP (vasoactive intestinal polypeptide). *Brain Research* 329:285, 1985.

(44) Goltman, A. M. The mechanism of migraine. *Journal of Allergy* 7:351, 1936.

(45) Graham, J. R. Cluster headache. *Headache* 11:175, 1972.

(46) Green, J. E. A survey of migraine in England, 1975–1976. *Headache* 17:67, 1977.

(47) Haas, D. C., and Sovner, R. D. Migraine attacks triggered by mild head trauma, and their relation to certain post-

traumatic disorders of childhood. *Journal of Neurology, Neurosurgery and Psychiatry* 32:548, 1969.

(48) Hanington, E.; Horn, M.; and Wilkinson, M. Further observations on the effects of tyramine, in *Background to Migraine*. Third Migraine Symposium. London: Heinemann, 1970, p. 113.

(49) Harris, W. Ciliary (migrainous) neuralgia and its treatment. *British Medical Journal* 1:57, 1936.

(50) Henderson, W. R., and Raskin, N. H. Hot-dog headache: Individual susceptibility to nitrite. *Lancet* 2:1162, 1972.

(51) Henryk-Gutt, R., and Rees, W. L. Psychological aspects of migraine. *Journal of Psychosomatic Research* 17:141, 1973.

(52) Horton, B. T.; MacLean, A. R.; and Craig, W. McK. A new syndrome of vascular headache: Results of treatment with histamine: Preliminary report. *Proceedings of Staff Meetings of Mayo Clinic* 14:257, 1939.

(53) Hubel, D. H., and Wiesel, T. N. Receptive fields and functional architecture of monkey striate cortex. *Journal of Physiology* (London) 195:215, 1968.

(54) Jacobson, E. *You Must Relax.* New York, Toronto, London: McGraw-Hill, 1962.

(55) Jannetta, P. J. Observations of the etiology of trigeminal neuralgia in 100 consecutive operative cases: Definitive microsurgical treatment by relief of compression-distortion of the trigeminal nerve at the brain stem. Paper delivered at the Neurosurgical Congress in Tokyo, Sept. 1973.

(56) Jones, J. *The Ice-Cream Headache and Other Stories.* London: Collins, 1968; Fontana Books, 1971.

(57) King, A. B., and Robinson, S. M. Vascular headaches of acute mountain sickness. *Aerospace Medicine*, August 1972, p. 849.

(58) Krabbe, A. A., and Olesen, J. Headache provocation by continuous intravenous infusion of histamine: Clinical results and receptor mechanisms. *Pain* 8:253, 1980.

(59) Kudrow, L. *Cluster Headache: Mechanisms and Management.* New York: Oxford University Press, 1980.

(60) Kunkle, E. C.; Pfeiffer, J. B.; Wilhoit, W. M.; and Lamrick, L. W. Recurrent brief headaches in "cluster" pattern. *North Carolina Medical Journal* 15:510, 1954.

(61) Lambert, G. A.; Bogduk, N.; Goadsby, P. J.; Duckworth, J. W.; and Lance, J. W. Decreased carotid arterial resistance in cats in response to trigeminal stimulation. *Journal of Neurosurgery* 61:307, 1985.

(62) Lance, J. W. Headaches related to sexual activity. *Journal of Neurology, Neurosurgery and Psychiatry* 39:1226, 1976.

(63) Lance, J. W. *Mechanism and Management of Headache,* fourth edition. London: Butterworths, 1982.

(64) Lance, J. W., and Anthony, M. Some clinical aspects of migraine. *Archives of Neurology* 15:356, 1966.

(65) Lance, J. W., and Anthony, M. Migrainous neuralgia or cluster headache? *Journal of Neurological Sciences* 13:401, 1971.

(66) Lance, J. W., and Anthony, M. Neck-tongue syndrome on sudden turning of the head. *Journal of Neurology, Neurosurgery and Psychiatry* 43:97, 1980.

(67) Lance, J. W., and Curran, D. A. Treatment of chronic tension headache. *Lancet* 1:1236, 1964.

(68) Lance, J. W.; Curran, D. A.; and Anthony, M. Investigations into the mechanism and treatment of chronic headache. *Medical Journal of Australia* 2:909, 1965.

(69) Lance, J. W.; Lambert, G. A.; Goadsby, P. J.; and Duckworth, J. W. Brainstem influences on the cephalic circulation: Experimental data from cat and monkey of relevance to the mechanism of migraine. *Headache* 23:258, 1983.

(70) Lashley, K. S. Patterns of cerebral integration indicated by the scotomas of migraine. *Archives of Neurology and Psychiatry* (Chicago) 46:331, 1941.

(71) Lee, C. H., and Lance, J. W. Migraine stupor. *Headache* 17:32, 1977.

(72) Lennox, W. G., and Lennox, M. A. *Epilepsy and Related Disorders,* Vol. 1. London: Churchill, 1960.

(73) Liveing, E. *On Megrim, Sick-Headache, and Some Allied Disorders: A Contribution to the Pathology of Nerve-Storms.* London: J. & A. Churchill, 1873.

(74) Loh, L.; Nathan, P. W.; Schott, G. D.; and Zilkha, K. J. Acupuncture versus medical treatment for migraine and muscle tension headaches. *Journal of Neurology, Neurosurgery and Psychiatry* 47:333, 1984.

(75) Martin, P. R., and Mathews, A. M. Tension headaches: Psycho-physiological investigations and treatment. *Journal of Psychosomatic Research* 22:389, 1978.

(76) Masters, W. H., and Johnson, V. E. *Human Sexual Response.* Boston: Little, Brown, & Co., 1966.

(77) Matthews, W. B. Footballer's migraine. *British Medical Journal* 1:326, 1972.

(78) McNally, W. *Smithy: The Kingsford Smith Story.* London: Robert Hale, 1966.

(79) Medina, J. L., and Diamond, S. The role of diet in migraine. *Headache* 18:31, 1978.

(80) Miller, H. Accident neurosis. *British Medical Journal*, Vol. 1, 1961.

(81) Mitchell, K. R., and Mitchell, D. M. Migraine: An exploratory treatment application of programmed behaviour therapy techniques. *Journal of Psychosomatic Research* 15:137, 1971.

(82) Moffett, A. M.; Swash, M.; and Scott, D. F. Effect of tyramine in migraine: A double-blind study. *Journal of Neurology, Neurosurgery and Psychiatry* 35:496, 1972.

(83) Moffett, A. M.; Swash, M.; and Scott, D. F. Effect of chocolate in migraine: A double-blind study. *Journal of Neurology, Neurosurgery and Psychiatry* 37:445, 1974.

(84) Monro, J.; Brostoff, J.; Carini, C.; and Zilkha, K. Food allergy in migraine: Study of dietary exclusion and RAST. *Lancet* 2:1, 1980.

(85) Moskowitz, M. A. The neurobiology of vascular head pain. *Annals of Neurology* 16:157, 1984.

(86) Olesen, J.; Larsen, B.; and Lauritzen, M. Focal hyperemia followed by spreading oligemia and impaired activation of rCBF in classical migraine. *Annals of Neurology* 9:344, 1981.

(87) Olesen, J.; Tfelt-Hansen, P.; Henricksen, L.; and Larsen, B. The common migraine attack may not be initiated by cerebral ischaemia. *Lancet* 2:438, 1981.

(88) Parker, G. B.; Tupling, H.; and Pryor, D. S. A controlled trial of cervical manipulation for migraine. *Australian and New Zealand Journal of Medicine* 8:589, 1978.

(89) Pearce, J. Insulin induced hypoglycaemia in migraine. *Journal of Neurology, Neurosurgery and Psychiatry* 34:154, 1971.

(90) Pestronk, A., and Pestronk, S. Goggle migraine. *New England Journal of Medicine* 308:226, 1983.

(91) Pope, A. *The Rape of the Lock.*

(92) Raskin, N. H., and Appenzeller, O. Headache, in *Major Problems in Internal Medicine*, Vol. 19, edited by J. H. Smith, Jr. Philadelphia: W. H. Saunders, 1980, p. 16.

(93) Raskin, N. H., and Knittle, S. C. Ice-cream headache and orthostatic symptoms in patients with migraine. *Headache* 16:222, 1976.

(94) Relander, M.; Troupp, H.; and Björkesten, G. Controlled trial of treatment for cerebral concussion. *British Medical Journal* 2:777, 1972.

(95) Rolf, L. H.; Wiele, G.; and Brune, G. G. 5-hydroxytryptamine in platelets of patients with muscle contraction headache. *Headache* 21:10, 1981.

(96) Romberg, M. H. *A Manual of Nervous Diseases of Man*, trans. by E. H. Sieveking. London: Sydenham Society, 1840.

(97) Rooke, E. D. Benign exertional headache. *Medical Clinics of North America* 52:801, 1968.

(98) Sachs, H.; Russell, J. A. G.; Christman, D. R.; Fowler, J. S.; and Wolf, A. P. Positron emission tomographic studies on induced migraine. *Lancet* 2:465, 1984.

(99) Schaumburg, H. H.; Byck, R.; Gerstl, R.; and Mashman, J. H. Monosodium L-glutamate: Its pharmacology and role in the Chinese restaurant syndrome. *Science* 163:826, 1969.

(100) Selby, G., and Lance, J. W. Observations on 500 cases of migraine and allied vascular headache. *Journal of Neurology, Neurosurgery and Psychiatry* 23:23, 1960.

(101) Sicuteri, F. Vasoneuroactive substances and their implication in vascular pain, in *Research and Clinical Studies in Headache*, Vol. 1. New York & Basel: Karger, 1967, p. 6.

(102) Sicuteri, F. Headache as possible expression of deficiency of brain 5-hydroxytryptamine: Central denervation supersensitivity. *Headache* 14:69, 1972.

(103) Sjaastad, O.; Apfelbaum, R.; Caskey, W.; Christoffersen, B.; Diamond, S.; Graham, J.; Green, M.; Hørven, I.; Lund-Roland, L.; Medina, J.; Rogado, S.; and Stein, H. Chronic paroxysmal hemicrania (CPH): The clinical manifestations —a review. *Uppsala Journal of Medical Sciences*, supplement 31, 1980, p. 27.

(104) Somerville, B. W. The role of progesterone in menstrual migraine. *Neurology* (Minneapolis) 21:853, 1971.

(105) Somerville, B. W. The role of estradiol withdrawal in the etiology of menstrual migraine. *Neurology* (Minneapolis) 22:355, 1972.

(106) Sulman, F. G. Serotonin-migraine in climatic heat stress: Its prophylaxis and treatment. *Proceedings of the International Headache Symposium*, Elsinore, Denmark, 1971. Basel: Sandoz Ltd., 1971, p. 45.

(107) Sulman, F. G.; Danon, A.; Pfeifer, Y.; Tal, E.; and Weller, C. P. Urinalysis of patients suffering from climatic heat stress (Sharav). *International Journal of Biometeorology* 14:205, 1970.

(108) Symonds, C. P. Cough headache. *Brain* 79:557, 1956.

(109) Taylor, A. R. Post-concussional sequelae. *British Medical Journal* 2:67, 1967.

(110) Tubbs, O. N., and Potter, J. M. Early post-concussional headache. *Lancet* 2:128, 1976.

(111) Walshe, F. Head injuries as a factor in the aetiology of intra-cranial meningioma. *Lancet* 2:993, 1961.

(112) Warner, G., and Lance, J. W. Relaxation therapy in migraine and chronic tension headache. *Medical Journal of Australia* 1:298, 1975.

(113) Weiss, E., and English, O. S. *Psychosomatic Medicine.* Philadelphia & London: W. B. Saunders, 1957.

(114) Wolff, H. G. *Headache and Other Head Pain.* New York: Oxford University Press, 1963.

INDEX

223